WITHERING ON THE FOXGLOVE AND OTHER CLASSICS IN PHARMACOLOGY

Edited with introductions by
LAWRENCE A. MAY, M.D.

distributed by
DABOR SCIENCE PUBLICATIONS
Oceanside, New York 11572

Introduction © 1977 by
Lawrence A. May

Library of Congress Cataloging in Publication Data
Main entry under title:

Withering, an account of the foxglove and other pharmacologic classics.

CONTENTS: Withering, W. An account of the foxglove.- -Sutton, Dr. and Want, J. Medical and philisophical intelligence.- -Brunton, T.L. On the use of nitrite of amyl in angina pectoris. [etc.]
    1. Chemotherapy- -Early works to 1800.   2. Angina pectoris- -Chemotherapy- -Early works to 1800.   3. Dropsy- -Chemotherapy- -Early works to 1800.   4. Rheumatism- -Chemotherapy- -Early works to 1800.   5. Digitalis- -Early works to 1800.   I. May, Lawrence A. II. Withering, William, 1741-1799. An account of the foxglove. 1977.
[DNLM: WZ292 W823]
RM263.W57 1977   615'.58   77-16180
ISBN 0-89561-056-6

A Milton Cohen Book

Printed in the United States of America

TABLE OF CONTENTS

INTRODUCTION

Pharmaceuticals are an essential part of the modern physician's therapeutic armamentarium. By our current standards of antibiotics, cancer chemotherapy, and psychotropic drugs, the pharmacologic efforts of our nineteenth-century predecessors seem primitive at best. In the 1800's, the principles of therapy involved bleeding, purgatives, blisters, and salts of heavy metals. We are reprinting a small collection of landmark articles in pharmacology which established the efficacy of drugs which are still relied on today by practicing physicians.

The monumental contribution to pharmacology in the eighteenth century was Withering's *Account of the Foxglove,* which we are reprinting in its entirety. William Withering was the most famous scion of a family of physicians. In 1776, he published a monograph on botany which, for many years, remained the standard botanical reference in Britain. He explains how he began using the foxglove for treating patients with edema:

> In the year 1775, my opinion was asked concerning a family receipt for the cure of the dropsy. I was told that it had long been kept a secret by an old woman in Shropshire, who had sometimes made cures after the more regular practitioners had failed. I was informed also, that the effects produced were violent vomiting

and purging; for the diuretic effects seemed to have been overlooked. This medicine was composed of twenty or more different herbs: but it was not very difficult for one conversant in these subjects, to perceive, that the active herb could be no other than the Foxglove.

Withering recognized many of the clinical implications of digitalis which we currently accept. He chose an appropriate dose of digitalis leaves, recognized the need for slow digitilization, and appreciated the danger of digitalis toxicity. His description of toxicity is valid today:

> I found him incessantly vomiting, his vision indistinct, his pulse 40 in a minute. On inquiry it came out that his wife had stewed a large handful of green Foxglove leaves in half a pint of water and given him the liquor which he drank at a draught in order to cure him of an asthmatic affection. This good woman knew the medicine of her county, but not the dose of it, for her husband narrowly escaped with his life.

Withering's account is a model of responsible reportage which, in its clear and well documented style, established the primacy of digitalis in treating disorders of volume overload.

Our second entry discusses the use of colchicine as the active agent in a popular therapy for gout. Colchicine, an alkaloid of colchicum autumnale (the autumn crocus), had been known since the sixth century when it was introduced by Alexander of Tralles. It was known to the Byzantines as hermodactyl. Colchicum was used extensively in patent medicines by charlatans, one of the best known being L'Eau d'Husson. Its benefit to gout sufferers was so unequivocal that efforts to remove the medicine were abandoned. Dr. Edwin Croddem Jones introduced the remedy to England and wrote a monograph about its use.

We are reprinting the important pharmacologic contribution of Dr. James Want in which he discusses his discovery that the basic ingredient of l'eau d'husson is clochicum. We are also reprinting the report of Dr. Want's work in which he speaks of the drug "producing nausea and loathing of food," a problem we still confront with colchicine. We have also reprinted Dr. Sutton's comments and Dr. Want's reply which illustrate the need for carefully controlled studies rather than dogmatic assertions. Want states in reply: "The identity of the tincture of colchicum and eau medicinale, is a question which can only be determined by attentive examination and comparison of their respective operations on the human body. Six years later, the alkaloid colchicine was isolated by the justly famous French chemists Pelletier and Caventou, who also isolated emetine and strychnine. Colchicine remains a specific and effective drug to treat gout.

The next two articles were landmarks in the therapy of angina pectoris. The first paper, by Brunton, on the use of amyl nitrite in angina pectoris is a classic extrapolation of experimental data to predict clinical effect. Brunton's laboratory work led him to recognize the elevation of blood pressure that accompanied angina and the blood pressure-reducing effect of nitrites. He writes:

From observations during the attack, and from an examination of numerous sphygmographic tracings taken while the patients were free from pain, while it was coming on, at its height, passing off under the influence of amyl, and again completely gone, I find that when the attack comes on gradually the pulse becomes smaller, and the arterial tension greater as the pain increases in severity. During the attack the breathing is quick, the pulse small and rapid, and the arterial tension high, owing, I believe, to contraction of the systemic capillaries. As the nitrite is inhaled the pulse becomes slower and fuller, the tension diminished, and the breathing less hurried.

Brunton's contributions were legion: he served as editor of the *Practitioner*, lectured on "materia medica," and authored a respected and widely used *Textbook of Pharmacology*. The paper we are reprinting is probably his most notable clinical contribution.

The next paper, written by William Murrell and published in 1879, suggests nitroglycerine as a remedy for angina pectoris. Murrell was a pharmacologist whose *Manual of Pharmacology and Therapeutics* was a widely used reference, and his book *What to Do in the Case of Poisoning* enjoyed eleven editions. In the paper we are reprinting, Murrell recognizes the adverse production of headache by nitroglycerine. His recommendation for the use of nitroglycerine derived from his appreciation that it exerts similar effects to amyl nitrite. He then points out the transitory effect of nitrites and writes, "The nitroglycerine produces its effect much more slowly, they last longer and disappear gradually, the tracing not resuming its normal condition for nearly half an hour." He concludes his paper by noting that the patient carried his medicine with him in a vial and used it when an attack seized him. He laconically comments, "It never failed to afford relief." Nearly one hundred years after Murrel's important paper, nitroglycerine remains an enormously effective drug.

The next article is Horace Green's report "On the Use and Effect of Applications of Nitrate of Silver to the Throat." Salts of heavy metals were in wide clinical use during Dr. Green's time. We chose to reprint his paper because it is scholarly, well referenced, and reflective of the time. Silver nitrate, though no longer used for all of the purposes which Green cites, remains an important topical agent. Today, silver nitrate is most frequently employed for the prophylaxis of gonococcal ophthalmia neonatorum. It is also in current use for cauterization and in styptic pencils to stop bleeding. Green was a prominent New York practitioner who wrote a classic *Treatise on Diseases of the Air Passages* and the historically interesting *Selections from Favorite Prescriptions of Living American Practitioners,* published in 1860. Green was a pugnacious American who served as Professor of Theory and Practice of Medicine at the New York Medical College. His self-confident approach is illustrated early in this important paper when he speaks about other works in his area of interest:

> These volumes contain nothing on this subject not recorded in my own work on *Diseases of the Air Passages,* published in 1846. I shall only allude to them in order to say, that however just the English may have been in accusing American writers of 'pirating' and of borrowing largely from English authors, they are themselves not altogether immaculate in this respect. One of these authors has taken copiously from the above work, without the ordinary acknowledgement; whilst the other has made up a good-looking volume of nearly two hundred

pages, on *Diseases of the Mucous Membrane of the Throat and their Treatment by Topical Medication*, a large proportion of which in its chapters on pathology, etiology and treatment, is abstracted from my work; page after page of matter having been copied literally, without any intimation whatever as to its true paternity, and that too without those revisions and improvements which might have been made advantageously with almost every sentence purloined.

The last article describes the use of salicin in the treatment of acute rheumatism by Thomas Maclagan. The willow bark, the source of salicin, was long known to have antipyretic qualities. In 1827, Leroux extracted a bitter glycoside called salicin. Sodium salicylate was used in 1875 as an antipyretic and for rheumatic fever by Buss. In the following year, Maclagan published the important paper that established the efficacy of salicylates in treating rheumatism. Maclagan was less a physiologist than he was a religious man who believed in the order of nature, and his description of what motivated his decision to use salicin contrasts with the scientific approach of the other papers we are reprinting:

> Impressed with this fact, and believing in the miasmatic origin of rheumatic fever, it seemed to me that a remedy for that disease would most hopefully be looked for among those plants and trees whose favourite habitat presented conditions analogous to those under which the rheumatic miasm seemed most to prevail. A low-lying, damp locality, with a cold, rather than warm, climate, give the conditions under which rheumatic fever is most readily produced. On reflection, it seemed to me that the plants whose haunts best corresponded to such a de-

scription were those belonging to the natural order Salicaceae, the various forms of willow.

Maclagan's scientific commitment is attested to by his restraint in not publishing his findings until he had accumulated a number of well documented cases. After Maclagan's paper, the German professor Herman Senator advocated the use of less toxic sodium salicylate, and, in 1899, Dreser introduced acetylsalicylate (aspirin), which has since been the main therapeutic agent for rheumatic diseases.

AN
ACCOUNT
OF THE
FOXGLOVE,
AND
Some of its Medical Uses:
WITH
PRACTICAL REMARKS ON DROPSY,
AND OTHER DISEASES.

BY

WILLIAM WITHERING, M. D.
Physician to the General Hospital at Birmingham.

———— nonumque prematur in annum.
HORACE.

BIRMINGHAM: PRINTED BY M. SWINNEY;
FOR
C. G. J. AND J. ROBINSON, PATERNOSTER-ROW, LONDON.
M,DCC,LXXXV.

PREFACE.

AFTER being frequently urged to write upon this subject, and as often declining to do it, from apprehension of my own inability, I am at length compelled to take up the pen, however unqualified I may still feel myself for the task.

The use of the Foxglove is getting abroad, and it is better the world should derive some instruction, however imperfect, from my experience, than that the lives of men should be hazarded by its unguarded exhibition, or that a medicine of so much efficacy should be condemned and rejected as dangerous and unmanageable.

It

It is now about ten years fince I firft began to ufe this medicine. Experience and
cautious attention gradually taught me how
to ufe it. For the laft two years I have not
had occafion to alter the modes of management; but I am ftill far from thinking
them perfect.

It would have been an eafy tafk to have
given felect cafes, whofe fuccefsful treatment
would have fpoken ftrongly in favour of the
medicine, and perhaps been flattering to my
own reputation. But Truth and Science
would condemn the procedure. I have
therefore mentioned every cafe in which I
have prefcribed the Foxglove, proper or improper, fuccefsful or otherwife. Such a
conduct will lay me open to the cenfure of
thofe who are difpofed to cenfure, but it
will meet the approbation of others, who are
the beft qualified to be judges.

To the Surgeons and Apothecaries, with
whom I am connected in practice, both in
this town and at a diftance, I beg leave to
make

make this public acknowledgment, for the
affiftance they fo readily afforded me, in per-
fecting fome of the cafes, and in communicating the events of others.

The ages of the patients are not always
exact, nor would the labour of making them
fo have been repaid by any ufeful confequences. In a few inftances accuracy in that
refpect was neceffary, and there it has been
attempted ; but in general, an approxima-
tion towards the truth, was fuppofed to be
fufficient.

The cafes related from my own experience, are generally written in the fhorteft
form I could contrive, in order to fave time
and labour. Some of them are given more
in detail, when particular circumftances
made fuch detail neceffary ; but the cafes
communicated by other practitioners, are
given in their own words.

I muft caution the reader, who is not a
practitioner in phyfic, that no general de-
ductions, decifive upon the failure or fuccefs

of the medicine, can be drawn from the cafes I now prefent to him. Thefe cafes muft be confidered as the moft hopelefs and deplorable that exift ; for phyficians are feldom confulted in chronic difeafes, till the ufual remedies have failed : and, indeed, for fome years, whilft I was lefs expert in the management of the Digitalis, I feldom prefcribed it, but when the failure of every other method compelled me to do it ; fo that upon the whole, the inftances I am going to adduce, may truly be confidered as cafes loft to the common run of practice, and only fnatched from deftruction, by the efficacy of the Digitalis; and this in fo remarkable a manner, that, if the properties of that plant had not been difcovered, by far the greateft part of thefe patients muft have died.

There are men who will hardly admit of any thing which an author advances in fupport of a favorite medicine, and I allow they may have fome caufe for their hefitation; nor do I expect they will wave their ufual modes of judg-

judging upon the prefent occafion. I could with therefore that fuch readers would pafs over what I have faid, and attend only to the communications from correfpondents, becaufe they cannot be fuppofed to poffefs any unjuft predilection in favour of the medicine: but I cannot advife them to this ftep, for I am certain they would then clofe the book, with much higher notions of the efficacy of the plant than what they would have learnt from me. Not that I want faith in the difcernment or in the veracity of my correfpondents, for they are men of eftablifhed reputation; but the cafes they have fent me are, with fome exceptions, too much felected. They are not upon this account lefs valuable in themfelves, but they are not the proper premifes from which to draw permanent conclufions.

I wifh the reader to keep in view, that it is not my intention merely to introduce a new diuretic to his acquaintance, but one which, though not infallible, I believe to be much more certain than any other in prefent ufe.

b 2

After

After all, in spite of opinion, prejudice, or error, TIME will fix the real value upon this discovery, and determine whether I have imposed upon myself and others, or contributed to the benefit of science and mankind.

Birmingham, 1*st July*, 1785.

INTRO-

INTRODUCTION.

THE Foxglove is a plant sufficiently common in this island, and as we have but one species, and that so generally known, I should have thought it superfluous either to figure or describe it; had I not more than once seen the leaves of Mullein* gathered for those of Foxglove. On the continent of Europe too, other species are found, and I have been informed that our species is very rare in some parts of Germany, existing only by means of cultivation, in gardens.

Our plant is the *Digitalis purpurea* † of Linnæus. It belongs to the 2d order of the 14th class, or the DIDYNAMIA ANGIOSPERMIA. The *essential characters* of the genus are, *Cup with 5 divisions. Blossom bell-shaped, bulging. Capsule egg-shaped, 2-celled.*— LINN.

DIGITA'LIS *purpu'rea.* Little leaves of the empalement egg-shaped, sharp. Blossoms blunt; the upper lip entire. LINN.

REFE-

---

* Verbascum of Linnæus.

† The trivial name *purpurea* is not a very happy one, for the blossoms though generally purple, are sometimes of a pure white.

References to Figures. Thefe are difpofed in the order of comparative excellence.

Rivini monopet. 104.
Flora danica, 74, *parts of fructification.*
Tournefort Inflitutiones. 73, *A, E, L, M.*
Fuchfii Hift. Plant. 893, *copied in*
Tragi ftirp. hiftor. 889.
J. Bauhini hiftor. Vol. ii. 812. 3, *and*
Lonicera 74, 1.
Blackwell. auct. 16.
Dodonæi pempt. ftirp. hift. 169, *reprinted in*
Gerard emacul. 790, 1, *and copied in*
Parkinfon Theatr. botanic. 653, 1.
Gerard, firft edition, 646, 1.
Hiftor. Oxon. Morifon. V. 8, *row* 1. 1.
Flor. danic. 74, *the reduced figure.*

Bloffom. The bellying part on the infide fprinkled with fpots like little eyes. *Leaves* wrinkled. Linn.

Blossom. Rather tubular than bell-fhaped, bulging on the under fide, purple; the narrow tubular part at the bafe, white. *Upper lip* fometimes flightly cloven.

Chives. *Threads* crooked, white. *Tips* yellow.

Pointal. *Seed-bud* greenifh. *Honey-cup* at its bafe more yellow. *Summit* cloven.

S. Vess. *Capfule* not quite fo long as the cup.

Root. Knotty and fibrous.

STEM.

STEM. About 4 feet high; obfcurely angular; leafy.

LEAVES. Slightly but irregularly ferrated, wrinkled; dark green above, paler underneath. *Lower leaves* egg-fhaped; upper leaves fpear-fhaped. *Leaf-ftalks* flefhy; bordered.

FLOWERS. Numerous, moftly growing from one fide of the ftem and hanging down one over another. *Floral-leaves* fitting, taper-pointed. The numerous purple bloffoms hanging down, mottled within; as wide and nearly half as long as the finger of a common-fized glove, are fufficient marks whereby the moft ignorant may diftinguifh this from every other Britifh plant; and the leaves ought not to be gathered for ufe but when the plant is in bloffom.

PLACE. Dry, gravelly or fandy foils; particularly on floping ground. It is a biennial, and flowers from the middle of *June* to the end of *July*.

I have not obferved that any of our cattle eat it. The root, the ftem, the leaves, and the flowers have a bitter herbaceous tafte, but I don't perceive that naufeous bitter which has been attributed to it.

This plant ranks amongft the LURIDÆ, one of the Linnæan orders in a natural fyftem. It has for congenera, NICOTIANA, ATROPA, HYOSCYAMUS, DATURA, SOLANUM, &c. fo that from the knowledge we poffefs of the virtues of thofe plants, and reafoning from botanical analogy, we might be led to guefs at fomething of its properties.

I in-

I intended in this place to have traced the history of its effects in diseases from the time of Fuchsius, who first describes it, but I have been anticipated in this intention by my very valuable friend, Dr. Stokes of Stourbridge, who has lately sent me the following

HISTORICAL VIEW of the Properties of Digitalis.

FUCHSIUS in his *hist. stirp.* 1542, is the first author who notices it. From him it receives its name of DIGITALIS, in allusion to the German name of *Fingerhut*, which signifies a finger-stall, from the blossoms resembling the finger of a glove.

SENSIBLE QUALITIES. Leaves bitterish, very nauseous. LEWIS *Mat. med.* i. 342.

SENSIBLE EFFECTS. Some persons, soon after eating of a kind of omalade, into which the leaves of this, with those of several other plants, had entered as an ingredient, found themselves much indisposed, and were presently after attacked with vomitings. DODONÆUS *pempt.* 170.

It is a medicine which is proper only for strong constitutions, as it purges very violently, and excites excessive vomitings. RAY. *hist.* 767.

BOERHAAVE judges it to be of a poisonous nature, *hist. plant.* but Dr. ALSTON ranks it among those indigenous vegetables, " which, though now disre-
" garded,

" garded, are medicines of great virtue, and fcarce-
" ly inferior to any that the Indies afford." LEWIS
Mat. med. i. *p.* 343.

Six or feven fpoonfuls of the decoction produce
naufea and vomiting, and purge: not without
fome marks of a deleterious quality. HALLER *hift. n.*
330 from *Aerial Inft. p.* 49, 50.

The following is an abridged ACCOUNT of
its EFFECTS upon TURKEYS.

M. SALERNE, a phyfician at Orleans, having heard
that feveral turkey pouts had been killed by being
fed with Foxglove leaves, inftead of mullein, he
gave fome of the fame leaves to a large vigorous
turkey. The bird was fo much affected that he
could not ftand upon his legs, he appeared drunk,
and his excrements became reddifh. Good nourifhment reftored him to health in eight days.

Being then determined to pufh the experiment
further, he chopped fome more leaves, mixed them
with bran, and gave them to a vigorous turkey cock
which weighed feven pounds. This bird foon appeared drooping and melancholy; his feathers ftared,
his neck became pale and retracted. The leaves
were given him for four days, during which time
he took about half a handful. Thefe leaves had
been gathered about eight days, and the winter was
far advanced. The excrements, which are naturally

ally green and well formed, became, from the first,
liquid and reddish, like those of a dysenteric patient.

The animal refusing to eat any more of this mixture which had done him so much mischief, I was
obliged to feed him with bran and water only; but
notwithstanding this, he continued drooping, and
without appetite. At times he was seized with convulsions, so strong as to throw him down; in the
intervals he walked as if drunk; he did not attempt
to perch, he uttered plaintive cries. At length he
refused all nourishment. On the fifth or sixth day
the excrements became as white as chalk; after-
terwards yellow, greenish, and black. On the eighteenth day he died, greatly reduced in flesh, for he
now weighed only three pounds.

On opening him we found the heart, the lungs,
the liver, and gall-bladder shrunk and dried up;
the stomach was quite empty, but not deprived of
its villous coat.   *Hist. de l'Academ.* 1748. *p.* 84.

EPILEPSY. — " It hath beene of later experience
" found also to be effectual against the falling sick-
" nesse, that divers have been cured thereby; for
" after the taking of the *Decoct. manipulor. ii. c. poly-.*
" *pod. quercin. contus.* ℥iv. *in cerevisia,* they that have
" been troubled with it twenty-six years, and have
" fallen once in a weeke, or two or three times in a
" moneth, have not fallen once in fourteen or fif-
" teen moneths, that is until the writing hereof."
                                    Parkinson, p. 654.
                                    SCROPHULA.—

SCROPHULA.—" The herb bruifed, or the juice
" made up into an ointment, and applied to the
" place, hath been found by late experience to be
" availeable for the King's Evill." PARK. p. 654.

Several hereditary inftances of this difeafe faid
to have been cured by it. AEREAL INFLUENCES, p
49, 50, quoted by HALLER, *hift. n.* 330.

A man with *fcrophulous ulcers* in various parts of
the body, and which in the right leg were fo viru-
lent that its amputation was propofed, cured by
*fucc. exprefs. cochl. i. bis intra xiv. dies, in ½ pinta
cerevifiæ calidæ.*

The leaves remaining after the preffing out of the
juice, were applied every day to the ulcers. *Pract.
efs. p. 40.* quoted by MURRAY *apparat medicam. i. p.*
491.

A young woman with a *fcrophulous tumour of the
eye,* a remarkable *fwelling of the upper lip, and painful
tumours of the joints of the fingers,* much relieved ;
but the medicine was left off, on account of its violent effects on the conftitution. *Ib. p.* 42 quoted as
above.

A man with a *fcrophulous tumour of the right elbow,*
attended for three years *with excruciating pains,* was
nearly cured by four dofes of the juice taken once
a month *Ib. p.* 43. as above.

The phyficians and furgeons of the Worcefter Infirmary have employed it in ointments and poul-
tices with remarkable efficacy. *Ib. p.* 44. It was re-
com-

commended to them by Dr. Baylies of Evesham, now of Berlin, as a remedy for this disease. Dr. Wall gave it a tryal, as well externally as internally, but their experiments did not lead them to observe any other properties in it, than those of a highly nauseating medicine and drastic purgative.

WOUNDS. In considerable estimation for the healing all kinds of wounds, *Lobel. adv.* 245.

Principally of use in ulcers, which discharge considerably, being of little advantage in such as are dry. HULSE, in R. hist. 768.

DOCTOR BAYLIES, physician to his Prussian Majesty, informed me, when at Berlin, that he employed it with great success in caries, and obstinate sore legs.

DYSPNŒA *Pituitosa* Sauvages i. 657.——" Boiled
" in water, or wine, and drunken doth cut and
" consume the thicke toughnesse of grosse, and
" slimie flegme, and naughtie humours. The
" same, or boiled with honied water or sugar, doth
" scoure and clense the brest, ripeneth and bring-
" eth foorth tough and clammie flegme. It open-
" eth also the stoppage of the liver spleene and
" milt, and of the inwarde parts." GERARDE hist.
" ed. I. p. 647.

" Whensoever there is need of a rarefying or
" extenuating of tough flegme or viscous humours
" troubling the chest,——the decoction or juice here-
" of made up with sugar or honey is availeable, as
" also to clense and purge the body both upwards
" and

" and downwards fometimes, of tough flegme, and
" clammy humours, notwithftanding that thefe
" qualities are found to bee in it, there are but few
" phyfitions in our times that put it to thefe ufes,
" but it is in a manner wholly neglected."

PARKINSON, p. 654.

Previous to the year 1777, you informed me of
the great fuccefs you had met with in curing dropfies by means of the fol. Digitalis, which you then
confidered as a more certain diuretic than any you
had ever tried. Some time afterwards, Mr. Ruffel,
furgeon, of Worcefter, having heard of the fuccefs which had attended fome cafes in which you
had given it, requefted me to obtain for him any
information you might be inclined to communicate
refpecting its ufe. In confeqnence of this application, you wrote to me in the following terms.*

In a letter which I received from you in London,
dated *September* 29, 1778, you write as follows:—
" I wifh it was as eafy to write upon the Digitalis—
" I defpair of pleafing myfelf or inftructing others,
" in a fubject fo difficult. It is much eafier to
" write upon a difeafe than upon a remedy. The
" former is in the hands of nature, and a faithful
" obferver, with an eye of tolerable judgment,
" cannot fail to delineate a likenefs. The latter
" will ever be fubject to the whims, the inaccura-
" cies, and the blunders of mankind."—

In

---

*: See the extract from this letter at page 5.

In my notes I find the following memorandum—
" *February* 20th, 1779, gave an account of Doctor
" Withering's practice, with the precautions ne-
" ceffary to its fuccefs, to the Medical Society at
" Edinburgh."—In the courfe of that year, the Di-
gitalis was prefcribed in the Edinburgh Infirmary, by
Dr. Hope, and in the following year, whilft I was
Clerk to Dr. Home, as Clinical Profeffor, I had a
favourable opportunity of obferving its fenfible ef-
fects.

In one cafe in which it was given properly at firft,
the urine began to flow freely on the fecond day.
On the third, the fwellings began to fubfide. The
dofe was then increafed more than *quadruple* in the
twenty-four hours. On the fifth day ficknefs came
on, and much purging, but the urine ftill increafed
though the pulfe funk to 50. On the 7th day, a
quadruple dofe of the infufion was ordered to be taken
every third hour, fo as to bring on naufea again.
The pulfe fell to forty-four, and at length to thirty-
five in a minute. The patient gradually funk and
died on the fixteenth day ; but previous to her
death, for two or three days, her pulfe rofe to near
one hundred.—It is needlefs to obferve to you, how
widely the treatinent of this cafe differed from the
method which you have found fo fuccefsful.

OF

OF THE PLATE.

THE figure of the Foxglove, facing the Title Page, is copied by the permiffion and under the infpection of Mr. Curtis, from his admirable work, entitled FLORA LONDINENSIS. The accuracy of the drawings, the beauty of the colouring, the full defcriptions, the accurate fpecific diftinctions, and the ufes of the different plants, cannot fail to recommend that work to the patronage of all who are interefted in the encouragement of genius, or the promotion of ufeful knowledge.

EXPLANATION.

Fig. 1. The Empalement.

Fig. 2, 3, 4. Four CHIVES two long and two fhort. TIPS at firft large, turgid, oval, touching at bottom, of a yellowifh colour, and often fpotted ; laftly changing both their form and fituation in a fingular manner.

Fig. 5, 6, 7. SEED-BUD rather conical, of a yellow green colour. *Shaft* fimple. *Summit* cloven.

Fig. 8. *Honeycup* a gland, furrounding the bottom of the Seed-bud.

Fig. 9. SEED-VESSEL, a pointed oval *Capfule*, of two cells and two valves, the lowermoft valve fplitting in two.

Fig. 10. SEEDS numerous, blackifh, fmall, lopped at each end.

AN

AN

A C C O U N T

OF THE

INTRODUCTION of FOXGLOVE

INTO

MODERN PRACTICE.

A S the more obvious and fenfible properties of
plants, fuch as colour, tafte, and fmell, have
but little connexion with the difeafes they are adapted
to cure; fo their peculiar qualities have no certain
dependence upon their external configuration. Their
chemical examination by fire, after an immenfe
wafte of time and labour, having been found ufe-
lefs, is now abandoned by general confent. Poffibly other modes of analyfis will be found out,
which may turn to better account; but we have hitherto made only a very fmall progrefs in the che-
miftry of animal and vegetable fubftances. Their
virtues muft therefore be learnt, either from obferving their effects upon infects and quadrupeds; from
analogy, deduced from the already known powers
of fome of their congenera, or from the empirical
ufages and experience of the populace.

The firft method has not yet been much attended
to; and the fecond can only be perfected in proportion as we approach towards the difcovery of a truly
natural fyftem; but the laft, as far as it extends, lies

A   within

within the reach of every one who is open to information, regardless of the source from whence it springs.

It was a circumstance of this kind which first fixed my attention on the Foxglove.

In the year 1775, my opinion was asked concerning a family receipt for the cure of the dropsy. I was told that it had long been kept a secret by an old woman in Shropshire, who had sometimes made cures after the more regular practitioners had failed. I was informed also, that the effects produced were violent vomiting and purging; for the diuretic effects seemed to have been overlooked. This medicine was composed of twenty or more different herbs; but it was not very difficult for one conversant in these subjects, to perceive, that the active herb could be no other than the Foxglove.

My worthy predecessor in this place, the very humane and ingenious Dr. Small, had made it a practice to give his advice to the poor during one hour in a day. This practice, which I continued until we had an Hospital opened for the reception of the sick poor, gave me an opportunity of putting my ideas into execution in a variety of cases; for the number of poor who thus applied for advice, amounted to between two and three thousand annually. I soon found the Foxglove to be a very powerful diuretic; but then, and for a considerable time afterwards, I gave it in doses very much too

large

large, and urged its continuance too long; for misled by reasoning from the effects of the squill, which generally acts best upon the kidneys when it excites nausea, I wished to produce the same effect by the Foxglove. In this mode of prescribing, when I had so many patients to attend to in the space of one, or at most of two hours, it will not be expected that I could be very particular, much less could I take notes of all the cases which occurred. Two or three of them only, in which the medicine succeeded, I find mentioned amongst my papers. It was from this kind of experience that I ventured to assert, in the Botanical Arrangement published in the course of the following spring, that the Digitalis purpurea " merited more attention than modern practice be- " stowed upon it."

I had not, however, yet introduced it into the more regular mode of prescription; but a circumstance happened which accelerated that event. My truly valuable and respectable friend, Dr. Ash, informed me that Dr. Cawley, then principal of Brazen Nose College, Oxford, had been cured of a Hydrops Pectoris, by an empirical exhibition of the root of the Foxglove, after some of the first physicians of the age had declared they could do no more for him. I was now determined to pursue my former ideas more vigorously than before, but was too well aware of the uncertainty which must attend on the exhibition of the *root* of a *biennial* plant, and therefore continued to use the *leaves*. These I had found to vary much as to dose, at different seasons of the year;

but I expected, if gathered always in one condition of the plant, viz. when it was in its flowering ſtate, and carefully dried, that the doſe might be aſcertained as exactly as that of any other medicine: nor have I been diſappointed in this expectation. The more I ſaw of the great powers of this plant, the more it ſeemed neceſſary to bring the doſes of it to the greateſt poſſible accuracy. I ſuſpected that this degree of accuracy was not reconcileable with the uſe of a *decoction*, as it depended not only upon the care of thoſe who had the preparation of it, but it was eaſy to conceive from the analogy of another plant of the ſame natural order, the tobacco, that its active properties might be impaired by long boiling. The decoction was therefore diſcarded, and the *infuſion* ſubſtituted in its place. After this I began to uſe the leaves in *powder*, but I ſtill very often preſcribe the infuſion.

Further experience convinced me, that the *diuretic* effects of this medicine do not at all depend upon its exciting a nauſea or vomiting; but, on the contrary, that though the increaſed ſecretion of urine will frequently ſucceed to, or exiſt along with theſe circumſtances, yet they are ſo far from being friendly or neceſſary, that I have often known the diſcharge of urine checked, when the doſes have been imprudently urged ſo as to occaſion ſickneſs.

If the medicine purges, it is almoſt certain to fail in its deſired effect; but this having been the caſe, I have ſeen it afterwards ſucceed when joined with
ſmall

small doses of opium, so as to restrain its action on
the bowels.

In the summer of the year 1776, I ordered a
quantity of the leaves to be dried, and as it then
became possible to ascertain its doses, it was gradually adopted by the medical practitioners in the circle of my acquaintance.

In the month of *November* 1777, in consequence
of an application from that very celebrated surgeon,
Mr. Russel, of Worcester, I sent him the following
account, which I choose to introduce here, as shew-
ing the ideas I then entertained of the medicine,
and how much I was mistaken as to its real dose.——
" I generally order it in decoction. Three drams of
" the dried leaves, collected at the time of the blof-
" soms expanding, boiled in twelve to eight ounces of
" water. Two spoonfuls of this medicine, given eve-
" ry two hours, will sooner or later excite a nausea.
" I have sometimes used the green leaves gathered in
" winter, but then I order three times the weight;
" and in one instance I used three ounces to a pint
" decoction, before the desired effect took place. I
" consider the Foxglove thus given, as the most cer-
" tain diuretic I know, nor do its diuretic effects
" depend merely upon the nausea it produces, for
" in cases where squill and ipecac. have been so
" given as to keep up a nausea several days together,
" and the flow of urine not taken place, I have found
" the Foxglove to succeed; and I have, in more than
" one instance, given the Foxglove in smaller and
A 3 " more

" more diftant dofes, fo that the flow of urine has
" taken place without any fenfible affection of the
" ftomach; but in general I give it in the manner
" firft mentioned, and order one dofe to be taken
" after the ficknefs commences. I then omit all me-
" dicines, except thofe of the cordial kind are wanted,
" during the fpace of three, four, or five days. By
" this time the naufea abates, and the appetite be-
" comes better than it was before. Sometimes the
" brain is confiderably affected by the medicine, and
" indiftinct vifion enfues; but I have never yet
" found any permanent bad effects from it."——

" I ufe it in the Afcites, Anafarca, and Hydrops
" Pectoris; and fo far as the removal of the water
" will contribute to cure the patient, fo far may be
" expected from this medicine: but I wifh it not to
" be tried in afcites of female patients, believing
" that many of thefe cafes are dropfies of the ovaria;
" and no fenfible man will ever expect to fee thefe
" encyfted fluids removed by any medicine."

" I have often been obliged to evacuate the water
" repeatedly in the fame patient, by repeating the
" decoction; but then this has been at fuch diftances
" of time as to allow of the interference of other
" medicines and a proper regimen, fo that the patient
" obtains in the end a perfect cure. In thefe cafes
" the decoction becomes at length fo very difagree-
" able, that a much fmaller quantity will produce the
" effect, and I often find it neceffary to alter its
" tafte by the addition of Aq. Cinnam. fp. or Aq.
" Juniper compofita."   " I al-

" I allow, and indeed enjoin my patients to drink
" very plentifully of fmall liquors through the whole
" courfe of the cure; and fometimes, where the eva-
" cuations have been very fudden, I have found a
" bandage as neceffary as in the ufe of the trochar."—

Early in the year 1779, a number of dropfical
cafes offered themfelves to my attention, the confequences of the fcarlet fever and fore throat which
had raged fo very generally amongft us in the preceding year. Some of thefe had been cured by
fquills or other diuretics, and relapfed; in others,
the dropfy did not appear for feveral weeks after the
original difeafe had ceafed: but I am not able to
mention many particulars, having omitted to make
notes. This, however, is the lefs to be regretted,
as the fymptoms in all were very much alike, and
they were all without an exception cured by the Foxglove.

This laft circumftance encouraged me to ufe the
medicine more frequently than I had done heretofore, and the increafe of practice had taught me to
improve the management of it.

In *February* 1779, my friend, Dr. Stokes, communicated to the Medical Society at Edinburgh the re-
fult of my experience of the Foxglove; and, in a letter addreffed to me in *November* following, he fays,
" Dr. Hope, in confequence of my mentioning its
" ufe to my friend, Dr. Broughton, has tried the
" Foxglove in the Infirmary with fuccefs." Dr.
Stokes

Stokes alſo tells me that Dr. Hamilton cured Dropſies with it in the year 1781.

I am informed by my very worthy friend Dr. Duncan, that Dr. Hamilton, who learnt its uſe from Dr. Hope, has employed it very frequently in the Hoſpital at Edinburgh. Dr. Duncan alſo tells me, that tne late very ingenious and accompliſhed Mr. Charles Darwin, informed him of its being uſed by his father and myſelf, in caſes of Hydrothorax, and that he has ever ſince mentioned it in his lectures, and ſometimes employed it in his practice.

At length, in the year 1783, it appeared in the new edition of the Edinburgh Pharmacopœia, into which, I am told, it was received in conſequence of the recommendation of Dr. Hope. But from which, I am ſatisfied, it will be again very ſoon rejected, if it ſhould continue to be exhibited in the unre-ſtrained manner in which it has heretofore been uſed at Edinburgh, and in the enormous doſes in which it is now directed in London.

In the following caſes the reader will find other diſeaſes beſides dropſies; particularly ſeveral caſes of conſumption. I was induced to try it in theſe, from being told, that it was much uſed in the Weſt of England, in the Phthiſis Pulmonalis, by the common people. In this diſeaſe, however, in my hands, it has done but little ſervice, and yet I am diſpoſed to wiſh it a further trial, for in a copy of Parkinſon's Herbal, which I ſaw about two years ago, I found

I found the following manuscript note at the article Digitalis, written, I believe, by a Mr. Saunders, who practised for many years with great reputation as a surgeon and apothecary at Stourbridge, in Worcestershire.

" Consumptions are cured infallibly by weak de-
" coction of Foxglove leaves in water, or wine and
" water, and drank for constant drink. Or take of
" the juice of the herb and flowers, clarify it, an
" make a fine syrup with honey, of which take
" three spoonfuls thrice in a day, at physical hours.
" The use of these two things of late has done, in
" consumptive cases, great wonders. But be cautious
" of its use, for it is of a vomiting nature. In
" these things begin sparingly, and increase the dose
" as the patient's strength will bear, least, instead of
" a sovereign medicine, you do real damage by this
" infusion or syrup."

The precautions annexed to his encomiums of this medicine, lead one to think that he has spoken from his own proper experience.

I have lately been told, that a person in the neighbourhood of Warwick, possesses a famous family receipt for the dropsy, in which the Foxglove is the active medicine; and a lady from the western part of Yorkshire assures me, that the people in her country often cure themselves of dropsical complaints by drinking Foxglove tea. In confirmation of this, I recollect about two years ago being desired to visit a
travelling

travelling Yorkſhire tradeſman. I found him inceſ-
ſantly vomiting, his viſion indiſtinct, his pulſe forty
in a minute. Upon enquiry it came out, that his
wife had ſtewed a large handſul of green Foxglove
leaves in half a pint of water, and given him the
liquor, which he drank at one draught, in order to
cure him of an aſthmatic affection. This good woman knew the medicine of her country, but not
the doſe of it, for her huſband narrowly eſcaped
with his life.

It is probable that this rude mode of exhibiting
the Foxglove has been more general than I am at
preſent aware of; but it is wonderful that no author
ſeems to have been acquainted with its effects as a
diuretic.

C A S E S,

C A S E S,

In which the Digitalis was given by the Direction of the Author.

1775.

IT was in the courfe of this year that I began to ufe the Digitalis in dropfical cafes. The patients were fuch as applied at my houfe for advice gratis. I cannot pretend to charge my memory with particular cafes, or particular effects, and I had not leifure to make notes. Upon the whole, however, it may be concluded, that the medicine was found ufeful, or I fhould not have continued to employ it.

C A S E I.

December 8th. A man about fifty years of age, who had formerly been a builder, but was now much reduced in his circumftances, complained to me of an afthma which firft attacked him about the latter end of autumn. His breath was very fhort, his countenance was funken, his belly large; and, upon examination, a fluctuation in it was very perceptible. His urine for fome time paft had been fmall in quantity. I directed a decoction of Fol. Digital. recent. which made him very fick, the ficknefs recurring at intervals for feveral days, during which time he made a large quantity of water. His breath gradually drew eafier, his belly fubfided, and in

about

about ten days he began to eat with a keen appetite. He afterwards took steel and bitters.

1776.

C A S E II.

January 14th. A poor man labouring under an afcites and anafarca, was directed to take a decoction of Digitalis every four hours. It purged him fmartly, but did not relieve him. An opiate was now ordered with each dofe of the medicine, which then acted upon the kidneys very freely, and he foon loft all his complaints.

C A S E III.

March 15th. A poor boy, about nine years of age, was brought for my advice. His countenance was pale, his pulfe quick and feeble, his body greatly emaciated, except his belly, which was very large, and, upon examination, contained a fluid. The cafe had been confidered as arifing from worms. He was directed to take the decoction of Digitalis night and morning. It operated as a diuretic, never made him fick, and he got well without any other medicine.

C A S E IV.

July 25th. Mrs. H———, of A———, near N———, between forty and fifty years of age, a few weeks ago, after fome previous indifpofition, was attacked by a fevere cold fhivering fit, fucceeded by fever: great pain in her left fide, fhortnefs of breath, perpetual cough, and, after fome days,

copious

copious expectoration. On the 4th of *June*, Dr.
Darwin,* was called to her. I have not heard what
was then done for her, but, between the 15th of *June*,
and 25th of *July*, the Doctor, at his different visits,
gave her various medicines of the deobstruent, tonic, antispasmodic, diuretic, and evacuant kinds.

On the 25th of *July* I was desired to meet Dr.
Darwin at the lady's house. I found her nearly in
a state of suffocation; her pulse extremely weak and
irregular, her breath very short and laborious, her
countenance sunk, her arms of a leaden colour,
clammy and cold. She could not lye down in bed,
and had neither strength nor appetite, but was extremely thirsty. Her stomach, legs, and thighs
were greatly swollen; her urine very small in quantity, not more than a spoonful at a time, and that
very seldom. It had been proposed to scarify her
legs, but the proposition was not acceded to.

She had experienced no relief from any means that
had been used, except from ipecacoanha vomits; the
dose of which had been gradually increased from 15
to 40 grains, but such was the insensible state of her
stomach for the last few days, that even those very
large doses failed to make her sick, and consequently purged her. In this situation of things I knew
of nothing likely to avail us, except the Digitalis:
but this I hesitated to propose, from an apprehension that little could be expected from any thing;
that an unfavourable termination would tend to
discredit

---

* Then resident at Lichfield, now at Derby.

difcredit a medicine which promifed to be of great
benefit to mankind, and I might be cenfured for a
prefcription which could not be countenanced by
the experience of any other regular practitioner.
But thefe confiderations foon gave way to the defire
of preferving the life of this valuable woman, and
accordingly I propofed the Digitalis to be tried;
adding, that I fometimes had found it to fucceed
when other, even the moft judicious methods, had
failed.   Dr. Darwin very politely, acceded immediately to my propofition, and, as he had never.
feen it given, left the preparation and the dofe to
my direction.   We therefore prefcribed as follows:

R. Fol. Digital. purp. recent. ʒiv. coque ex
   Aq. fontan. puræ ℔ifs ad ℔i. et cola.
R. Decoct. Digital. ʒifs.
   Aq. Nuc. Mofchat. ʒii. M. fiat. hauft. 2dis
horis fumend.

The patient took five of thefe draughts, which
made her very fick, and acted very powerfully upon the kidneys, for within the firft twenty-four
hours fhe made upwards of eight quarts of water.
The fenfe of fulnefs and oppreffion acrofs her ftomach was greatly diminifhed, her breath was eafed,
her pulfe became more full and more regular, and
the fwellings of her legs fubfided.

26th. Our patient being thus fnatched from impending deftruction, Dr. Darwin propofed to give
her a decoction of pareira brava and guiacum fhav-
                                                ings.

ings, with pills of myrrh and white vitriol; and, if coſtive, a pill with calomel and aloes. To theſe propoſitions I gave a ready aſſent.

30th. This day Dr. Darwin ſaw her, and directed a continuation of the medicines laſt preſcribed.

Auguſt 1ſt. I found the patient perfectly free from every appearance of dropſy, her breath quite eaſy, her appetite much improved, but ſtill very weak. Having ſome ſuſpicion of a diſeaſed liver, I directed pills of ſoap, rhubarb, tartar of vitriol, and calomel to be taken twice a day, with a neutral ſaline draught.

9th. We viſited our patient together, and repeated the draughts directed on the 26th of *June*, with the addition of tincture of bark, and alſo ordered pills of aloes, guiacum, and ſal martis to be taken if coſtive.

September 10th. From this time the management of the caſe fell entirely under my direction, and perceiving ſymptoms of effuſion going forwards, I deſired that a ſolution of merc. ſubl. corr. might be given twice a day.

19th. The increaſe of the dropſical ſymptoms now made it neceſſary to repeat the Digitalis. The dried leaves were uſed in infuſion, and the water was preſently evacuated, as before.

It

It is now almoſt nine years ſince the Digitalis was firſt preſcribed for this lady, and notwithſtanding I have tried every preventive method I could deviſe, the dropſy ſtill continues to recur at times ; but is never allowed to increaſe ſo as to cauſe much diſ-treſs, for ſhe occaſionally takes the infuſion and re-lieves herſelf whenever ſhe chooſes. Since the firſt exhibition of that medicine, very ſmall doſes have been always found ſufficient to promote the flow of urine.

I have been more particular in the narrative of this caſe, partly becauſe Dr. Darwin has related it ra-ther imperfectly in the notes to his ſon's poſthumous publication, truſting, I imagine, to memory, and partly becauſe it was a caſe which gave riſe to a ve-ry general uſe of the medicine in that part of Shrop-ſhire.

C A S E V.

December 10th. Mr. L———, Æt. 35. Aſcites and anaſarca, the conſequence of very intemperate living. After trying ſquill and other medicines to no purpoſe, I directed a decoction of the Fol. Digi-tal. recent. ſix drams to a pint; an eighth part to be taken every fourth hour. This made him ſick, and produced a copious flow of urine, but not enough to remove all the dropſical ſymptoms. After a fort-night a ſtronger decoction was ordered, and, upon a third trial, as the winter advanced, it became neceſſary to uſe four ounces to the pint decoction; and thus he got free from all his complaints.

In

In *October* 1777, in confequence of having purfued his intemperate mode of living, his dropfy returned, accompanied by evident marks of difeafed
vifcera. A decoction of two drams of Fol. Digital.
ficcat. to a pint, once more removed the dropfy. He
took a wine glafs full thrice a day.

In *January* 1778, I was defired to vifit him again.
I found he had gone on in his ufual intemperate life,
his countenance jaundiced, and the dropfy coming
on apace. After giving fome deobftruent medicines, I again directed the Digitalis, which again
emptied the water; but he did not furvive many
weeks.

1777.

C A S E   VI.

February —. Mrs. M———, Æt. 45. Afcites
and anafarca, but not much otherwife difeafed, and
well enough to walk about the houfe, and fee after
her family affairs. I thought this a fair cafe for a
trial of the Digitalis, and therefore directed a decoction of the frefh leaves, the ftock of dried ones
being exhaufted. About a week afterwards, calling
to fee my patient, I was informed that fhe was dead;
that the third day after my firft vifit fhe fuddenly
fell down, and expired. Upon enquiry I found
fhe had not taken any of the medicine; for the
fnow had lain fo deep upon the ground, that the
apothecary had not been able to procure it. Had

B   the

the medicine been given in a cafe feemingly fo favourable as this, and had the patient died under its
ufe, is it not probable that the death would have
been attributed to it?

C A S E   VII.

February 11th. Mr. E——, of W——, Æt. 61.
Hydrothorax, afcites and anafarca, confequences of
hard drinking.   He had been attended for fome
time by a phyfician in his neighbourhood, who had
treated his cafe with the ufual remedies. but without affording him any relief; nor could I expect to
fucceed better by any other medicine than the Digitalis.   The dried leaves were not to be had; and
the green ones at this feafon being very uncertain in
their ftrength,   I ordered four ounces of the roots
in a pint decoction, and directed three fpoonfuls to
be given every fourth hour, until it either excited
naufea, or a free difcharge of urine; both thefe
effects took place nearly at the fame time: he made
a large quantity of water, the fwellings fubfided
very confiderably, and his breath became eafy. Eight
days afterwards he began upon a courfe of bitters
and deobftruents.   The dropfical fymptoms foon
increafed again, but he had fuffered fo much from
the feverity of the ficknefs before, that he was neither willing to take, nor I to give the fame medicine
again.

Perhaps this patient might have been faved, if I
had been well acquainted with the management and
real

real doſes of the medicine, which was certainly in
this inſtance made very much too ſtrong; and notwithſtanding the caution to ſtop the further exhibition
when certain effects ſhould take place, it ſeems the
quantity previouſly ſwallowed was ſufficient to diſtreſs
him exceedingly.

C A S E   VIII.

March 11th. Mrs. H————, Æt. 32. A few
days after a tedious labour, had her legs and thighs
ſwelled to a very great degree; pale and ſemi-tranſ-
parent,* with pain in both groins. After a purge of
calomel and rhubarb, ung. merc. was ordered to be
rubbed upon the groins, and the following decoction
was directed:

R. Fol. Digital. purp. recent. ʒii.
 Aq. puræ. ℔i. coque ad ℔iſs et colatur. adde.
 Aq. cinn. ſp. ʒiv. M. capiat. cyath. vinos.
parv. bis quotidie.

The decoction preſently increaſed the ſecretion
of urine, and abated the diſtenſion of the legs: in
a fortnight the ſwelling was gone; but ſome days
after leaving her bed, her legs ſwelled again about
the ancles, which was removed by another bottle
of the decoction on the 21ſt of *April.*

---

* This diſeaſe has lately been well deſcribed by Mr. White,
of Mancheſter.

C A S E   IX.

March 29th.   Mr. G———, Æt. 47.   Very much deformed; afthma of feveral years continuance, but now dropfical to a great degree.   Took feveral medicines without relief, and then tried the Digitalis, but with no better fuccefs.

C A S E   X.

April 10th.   G—G———, Æt. 70.   Afthma and anafarca.   Took a decoction of the frefh leaves of the Digitalis, which produced violent ficknefs, but no immediate evacuation of water.   After the ficknefs had ceafed altogether, the urine began to flow copioufly, and he was cured.

C A S E   XI.

July 10th.   Mr. M——— of T———, Æt. 54.   A very hard drinker; had been affected fince *November* laft with afcites and anafarca, for which he had taken feveral medicines without benefit.   A decoction of the recent leaves of the Digitalis was then directed, an ounce and half to a pint, one eighth of which I ordered to be given every fourth hour. A few dofes brought on great naufea, indiftinct vifion, and a great flow of urine, fo as prefently to empty him of all the dropfical water.   Indeed the evacuation was fo rapid and fo complete, that it became neceffary to apply a bandage round the belly, and to fupport him with cordials.

In fomething more than a year and a half, his dropfy returned, but the Digitalis did not then fucceed to our wifhes. In *Auguft*, 1779, he was tapped, and lived afterwards only about five weeks.

For more particulars, fee the extract of a letter from Mr. Lyon.

C A S E   XII.

September 12th. Mifs C—— of T——, Æt. 48. An ovarium dropfy, and anafarcous legs and thighs. For three months in the beginning of this year fhe had been under the care of Dr. Darwin, who at different times had given her blue vitriol, elaterium, and calomel; decoction of pareira brava, and guiacum wood, with tincture of cantharides ; oxymel of. fquills, decoction of parfley roots, &c. Finding no relief, fhe difcontinued the ufe of medicines, until the urgency of her fymptoms induced her to afk my advice about the end of *Auguft*. She was greatly emaciated, and had almoft a total lofs of appetite. I firft tried fmall dofes of Merc. fublim. corr. in folution, with decoction of burdock roots, and blifters to the thighs. No advantage attending the ufe of this plan, I directed a decoction of Fol. Digit. a dram and half to a pint; one ounce to be taken twice a day. It prefently reduced the anafarcous fwellings, but made no alteration in the diftenfion of the abdomen.

CASE

C A S E XIII.

October 9th. Mrs. B——, Æt. 40. An ovarium dropfy. Took a decoction of Digitalis without effect. Her life was preferved for fome years by repeated tapping.

1778.

C A S E XIV.

February 8th. Mr. R—— of K——. Had formerly fuffered much from gout, and lived very intemperately. Jaundiced countenance; afcites; legs and thighs greatly fwollen; appetite none; extremely weak; confined to his bed. Had taken many medicines from his apothecary without advantage. I ordered him decoction of Digitalis, and a cordial; but he furvived only a few days.

C A S E XV.

March 13th. Mr. M——, Æt. 54. A thorax greatly deformed; afthma through the winter, fucceeded by dropfy in belly and legs. Pulfe very fmall; face leaden coloured; cough almoft continual. Decoction of feneka was directed, and fmall dofes of Dover's powder at night.

17th. Gum-ammoniac and fquill, with elixir paregor. at night —26th, Squill and decoction of feneka.—30th, His complaints ftill increafing, decoction

coction of Digitalis was then directed, which relieved him in a few days: but his complaints returned again, and he died in the month of *June*.

C A S E   XVI.

August 18th.   Mr. B——, Æt. 33.   Pulmonary confumption and dropfy.   The Digitalis, and that failing, other diuretics were ufed, in hopes of gaining fome relief from the diftrefs occafioned by the dropfical fymptoms; but none of them were effectual.   He was then attended by another phyfician, and died in about two months.

C A S E   XVII.

September 21ft.   Mrs. M—— W—— G——, Æt. 50.   An ovarium dropfy.   She took half a pint of Infuf. Digitalis, which made her fick, but did not increafe the quantity of urine.   She was afterwards relieved by tapping.

C A S E   XVIII.

October 28th.   R—— W——, Æt. 33.   Afcites and univerfal anafarca; countenance quite pale and bloated; appetite none, and the little food he forces down is generally rejected.

R. Fol. Digit. purp. ficcat. ʒiii.
    Aq. bull. ℔i. digere per horas duas, et colat. adde aq. junip. comp. ʒiii.

He

He was directed to take one ounce of this infusion
every two hours until it should make him sick.
This was on Wednesday. The fifth dose made
him vomit. On Thursday afternoon he vomited
again very freely, without having taken any more
of the medicine. On Friday and Saturday he made
more water than he had done for a week before,
and the swellings of his face and body were considerably abated. He was directed to omit all medicine so long as the urine continued to flow freely,
and also to keep an account of the quantity he made
in twenty-four hours.

These were his reports:

October 31st.	Saturday,	5 half pints.
November 1st.	Sunday,	6
2d.	Monday,	8
3d.	Tuesday,	8
4th.	Wednesday,	7
5th.	Thursday,	8

On Wednesday he began to purge, and the
purging still continues, but his appetite is better
than he has known it for a long time. No swelling
remains but about his ancles, extending at night
half way up his legs.

Omit all medicines at present.

7th.	Saturday,	7½ half pints.
8th.	Sunday,	8
9th.	Monday,	6¼
10th.	Tuesday,	6½
11th.	Wednesday,	6
12th.	Thursday,	6¼

On

On Tuesday the 17th, some swelling still remained about his ancles, but he was in every other respect perfectly well.

He took a few more doses of the infusion, and no other medicine.

C A S E XIX.

December 8th. W——— B———, Æt. 60. A hard drinker. Diseased viscera; ascites and anasarca. An infusion of Digitalis was directed, but it had no other effect than to make him sick.

1779.

In the beginning of this year we had many dropsies in children, who had suffered from the Scarlatina Anginosa; they all yielded very readily to the Digitalis, but in some the medicine purged, and then it did not prove diuretic, nor did it remove the dropsy until opium was joined with it, so as to prevent it purging. ———I did not keep notes of these cases, but I do not recollect a single instance in which the Digitalis failed to effect a cure.

C A S E XX.

January 1st. Mr. H———. Hydrops Pectoris; legs and thighs prodigiously anasarcous; a very distressing sense of fulness and tightness across his stomach; urine in small quantity; pulse intermitting; breath very short.

He

He had taken various medicines, and been blif-
tered, but without relief. His complamts continuing to increafe. I directed an infufion of Digitalis,
wiuch made him very fick; acted powerfully as a
diuretic, and removed all his fymptoms.

About three months afterwards he was out upon
a journev, and, after taking cold, was fuddenly
feized with difficulty of breathing, and violent palpitation of his heart: he fent for me, and I ordered
the infufion as before, which very foon removed
his complaints. He is now active and well; but,
whenever he takes cold, finds fome return of difficult
breathing, which he foon removes by a dofe or two
of the infufion.

C A S E XXI.

January 5th. Mrs. M——, Æt. 69. Hydrothorax, (called afthma) afcites and anafarca. I directed an infufion of Fol. Digital. ficcat. three drams
to a pint; a fmall wine glafs to be taken every third
or fourth hour. It made her violently fick, acted
powerfully as a diuretic, fet her breath perfectly at
liberty, and carried off the fwelling of her legs;
when fhe was nearly emptied, fhe became fo languid, that I thought it neceffary to order cordials,
and a large blifter to her back. Mr. Ward, who
attended as her apothecary, tells me fhe had fome
return of her afthma in *June* and *October* following,
which was each time removed by the fame medicine.

CASE

C A S E XXII.

January 11th. Mr. H——, Æt. 59. Afcites and general anafarca. A large corpulent man, and a hard drinker: he had repeatedly fuffered under complaints of this kind, but had been always relieved by the judicious affiftance of Dr. Afh. In the prefent inftance, however, not finding relief as ufual from the prefcriptions of my worthy friend, he fent for me; after examining into his fituation, and informing myfelf what had been done to relieve him, I was fatisfied that the Digitalis was the only medicine from which I had any thing to hope. It was therefore directed; but another patient requiring my affiftance at a diftance from town, I defired he would not begin the medicine before I returned, which would be early on the third day; for I was well aware of the difficulties before me, and that he would inevitably fink under too rapid an evacuation of the water. On my return I was informed, that the preceding evening, as he fat on his chair, his head funk upon his breaft, and he died.

This cafe, as well as cafe VI. is mentioned with a view to demonftrate to younger practitioners, how fudden and unexpected the deaths of dropfical patients fometimes happen, and how cautious we fhould be in affigning caufes for effects.

C A S E XXIII.

Auguft 31ft. Mr. C——, Æt. 57. Difeafed vifcera, jaundice, afcites and anafarca. After trying

ing calomel, faline draughts, jallap purges, chryftals
of tartar, pills of gum ammoniac, fquills, and
foap, fal fuccini, eleterium, &c. infufion of Digitalis was directed, which removed all his urgent
fymptoms, and he recovered a pretty good ftate of
health.

C A S E XXIV.

September 11th. I was defired to vifit Mr. L——,
Æt. 63; a middle fized man; rather thin; not ha-
bitually intemperate; found him in bed, where he
had been for three days. He was in a ftate of furi-
ous infanity, and had been gradually lofing his reafon for ten days before, but was not outrageous the
firft week: his apothecary had given him ten grains
of emetic tartar, a dram of ipecacoanha, and an
ounce of tincture of jallap, in the fpace of a few
hours, which fcarcely made him fick, and only occafioned a ftool or two; upon enquiring into the
ufual ftate of his health, I was told that he had been
troubled with fome difficulty of breathing for thirty
years paft, but for the nine laft years this complaint
had increafed, fo that he was often obliged to fit up
the greater part of the night; and, for the laft year,
the fenfe of fuffocation was fo great, when he lay
down, that he often fat up for a week together. His
father died of an afthma before he was fifty. A few
years ago, at an election, where he drank more
than ufual, his head was affected as now, but in a
flighter degree, and his afthmatic fymptoms vanifhed; and now, notwithftanding he has been feveral
days

days in bed, he feels not the least difficulty in breathing.

Apprehending that the infanity might be owing to the fame caufe which had heretofore occafioned the afthma, and that this caufe was water; I ordered a decoction of the Fol. ficcat Digital. three drams to half a pint; three fpoonfuls to be taken every third hour: the fourth dofe made him fick; the medicine was then ftopped; the ficknefs continued at intervals, more or lefs, for four days, during which time he made a great quantity of water, and gradually became more rational. On the fifth day his appetite began to return, and the ficknefs ceafed, but the flow of urine ftill continued.

A week afterwards I faw him again, and examined him particularly; his head was then perfectly rational, apetite very good, breath quite eafy, permitting him to lie down in bed without inconvenience, makes plenty of water, coughs a little, and expectorates freely. He took no other medicine, except a little rhubarb when coftive.

C A S E XXV.

September 15th. Mr. J. R——, Æt. 50. Subject to an afthmatical complaint for more than twenty years, but was this year much worfe than ufual, and fymptoms of dropfy appeared In *July* he took G. ammon. fquill and feneka, with infuf. amarum and foffil alkaly. In *Auguft*, infufum amar.
with

with vin. chalyb. and at bed-time pil. ſtyr. and
ſquill. His complaints increaſing, the ſquill was
puſhed as far as could be borne, but without any
good effect. *September* 15th, an infuſion of Digitalis
was directed, but he died the next morning.

C A S E XXVI.

September 18th. Mrs. R——, Æt. 30. After a
ſevere child-bearing, found both her legs and thighs
ſwelled to the utmoſt ſtretch of the ſkin. They
looked pale, and almoſt tranſparent. The caſe being ſimilar to that related at No. VIII. I determined
upon a ſimilar method of treatment; but as this patient had an inflammatory ſore throat alſo, I wiſhed
to get that removed firſt, and in three or four days
it was done. I then directed an infuſion of Digitalis, which ſoon increaſed the urinary ſecretion,
and reduced the ſwellings, without any diſturbance
of her ſtomach.

A few days after quitting her bed and coming
down ſtairs, ſome degree of ſwelling in her legs returned, which was removed by calomel, an opening
electuary, and the application of rollers.

C A S E XXVII.

October 7th. Mr. F——, a little man, with a
ſpine and thorax greatly deformed; for more than
a year paſt had complained of difficult reſpiration,
and a ſenſe of fulneſs about his ſtomach; theſe complaints increaſing, his abdomen gradually enlarged,
and

and a fluctuation in it became perceptible. He had
no anasarca, no appearance of diseased viscera, and
no great paucity of urine. Purges and diuretics of
different kinds affording him no relief, my assistance
was desired. After trying squill medicines without
effect, he was ordered to take Pulv. fol. Digital. in
small doses. These producing no sensible effect,
the doses were gradually increased until nausea was
excited; but there was no alteration in the quantity
of urine, and consequently no relief to his complaints. I then advised tapping, but he would not
hear of it; however, the distress occasioned by the
increasing fulness of his belly at length compelled
him to submit to the operation on the 20th of November. It was necessary to draw off the water again
upon the following days:

> December the 8th.
> — — 27th.
> 1780. February the 4th.
> — — 23d.
> March the 9th.

During the intervals, no method I could think of
was omitted to prevent the return of the disease;
but nothing seemed to avail. In the operation of
February 23d, his strength was so much reduced,
that the water was not entirely removed; and on
the 9th of March, before his belly was half emptied, notwithstanding the most judicious application
of bandage, his debility was so great, that it was
judged prudent to stop. After being placed in bed,
the faintness and sickness continued; severe rigors
ensued,

enfued, and violent vomiting; thefe vomitings continued through the night, and in the intervals he
lay in a ftate nearly approaching to fyncope. The
next day I found him with nearly the fame fymptoms; but remarked that the quantity of fluid he
had thrown up was very much more than what he
had taken, and that his abdomen was confiderably
fallen; in the courfe of two or three days more, he
difcharged the whole of the effufed fluid; his ftrength
and appetite gradually returned, and he was in all
refpects much better than he had been before the
laft operation.

Some time afterwards, his belly began to fill
again, and he again applied to me; upon an accurate examination, I judged the quantity of fluid
might then be about four or five quarts. Nature
had pointed out the true method of cure in this
cafe; I therefore ordered him to bed, and directed
ipecacoanha vomits to be given night and morning
in two or three days the whole of the water was
removed by vomiting, for he never purged, nor
was the quantity of his urine increafed; his appetite and ftrength gradually returned; he never had
any further relapfe, and is now an active healthy
man. I muft leave the reader to make his own re-
flections on this fingular cafe.

CASE

1780.

C A S E XXVIII.

January 11th. Captain V——, Æt. 42. Had
suffered much from residing in hot climates, and
drinking very freely, particularly rum in large quantity. He had tried many physicians before I saw
him, but nothing relieved him. I found him
greatly emaciated, his countenance of a brownish
yellow; no appetite, extremely low, distressing
fulness across his stomach; legs and thighs greatly
swollen; pulse quick, and very feeble; urine in
small quantity. As he had evidently only a few
days to live, I ordered him nothing but a solution
of sal diureticus in cinnamon water, slightly acidu-
lated with syrup of lemons. This medicine effecting no change, and his symptoms becoming daily
more distressing, I directed an infusion of Digitalis.
A few doses occasioned a copious flow of urine,
without sickness or any other disturbance. The medicine was discontinued; and the next day the urine
continuing to be secreted very plentifully, he lost
his most distressing complaints, was in great spirits,
and ate a pretty good dinner. In the evening, as
he was conversing chearfully with some friends, he
stooped forwards, fell from his chair, and died instantly. Had he been in bed, I think there is reason to believe this fatal syncope, if such it was,
would not have happened.

C   CASE

C A S E   XXIX.

February 6th.   Mr. H——, Æt. 63.   A corpulent man; had suffered much from gout, which for the last year or two had formed very imperfectly. He had now symptoms of water in his chest, his belly and his legs.   An infusion of Digitalis removed these complaints, and after being confined for the greater part of the winter, he was well enough to get abroad again.   In the course of a month the dropsical symptoms returned, and were again removed by the same medicine.   Bitters and tonics were now occasionally prescribed. but his debility gradually increased, and he died some time afterwards; but the dropsy never returned.

C A S E   XXX.

February 17th.   Mr. D————, Æt. 50.   Ascites and anasarca, with symptoms of phthisis.   He had been a very hard drinker.   The infusum Digitalis removed his dropsical symptoms, and he was sufficiently recovered to take a journey; but as the spring advanced, the consumptive symptoms increased, and he died soon afterwards, perfectly emaciated.

C A S E   XXXI.

March 5th.   I was desired to visit Mrs. H——, a very delicate woman, who after a severe lying-in, had her legs and thighs swollen to a very great degree;

gree; pale and semi-transparent. I found her extremely faint, her pulse very small and slow; vomiting violently, and frequently purging. She was attended by a gentleman who had seen me give the Digitalis in a similar case of swelled legs after a lying-in (see Case XXVI.) about six months before. He had not considered that this patient was delicate, the other robust; nor had he attended to stop the exhibition of the medicine when its effects began to take place. The great distress of her situation was evidently owing to the imprudent and unlimited use of the Digitalis. I was very apprehensive for her safety; ordered her cordials and volatiles; a free supply of wine, chamomile tea with brandy for common drink, and blisters. The next day the situation of things was much the same, but with all this disturbance no increased secretion of urine. The same methods were continued; an opiate ordered at night, and liniment. volatile upon flannel applied to the groins, as she now complained of great pain in those parts. The third day the nausea was less urgent, the vomitings less frequent, the pulse not so slow. Camphorated spirit, with caustic volatile alkaly, .was applied to the stomach, emulsion given for common drink, and the same medicines repeated. From this time, the intervals became gradually longer between the fits of vomiting, the flow of urine increased, the swellings subsided, the appetite returned, and she recovered perfectly.

CASE

C A S E XXXII.

March 16th. Mr. D——, Æt. 70. A paralytic ſtroke had for ſome weeks paſt impaired the uſe of his left ſide, and he complained much of his breath, and of a ſtraitneſs acroſs his ſtomach; at length, an anaſarca and aſcites appearing, I had no doubt as to the cauſe of the former ſymptoms; but, upon account of his advanced age, and the paralytic affection, I heſitated to give the Digitalis, and therefore tried the other uſual modes of practice, until at length his breath would not permit him to lie down in bed, and his other ſymptoms increaſed ſo rapidly as to threaten a ſpeedy diſſolution. In this dilemma I ventured to preſcribe an infuſion of the Fol. ſiccat. Digital. which preſently excited a copious flow of urine, and made him very ſick; a ſtrong infuſion of chamomile flowers, with brandy, relieved the ſickneſs, but the diuretic effects of the Digitalis continuing, his dropſy was removed, and his breathing became eaſy. The palſy remained nearly in the ſaine ſtate. He lived until *Auguſt* 1782, and without any return of the dropſy.

C A S E XXXIII.

March 18th. Miſs S——, Æt. 5. Hydrocephalus internus. As the caſe did not yield to calomel, when matters were nearly advanced to extremities, it occurred to me to try the Infuſum Digitalis; a few doſes of which were given, but had no ſenſible effect.

CASE

C A S E XXXIV.

March 19th. A young lady, foon after the birth of an illegitimate child, became infane. After being near a month under my care, fwellings of her legs, which at firft had been attributed to weaknefs, extended to her thighs and belly; her urine became foul, and fmall in quantity, and the infanity remained nearly the fame. As it had been very difficult to procure evacuations by any means, I ordered half an ounce of Fol. Digital. ficcat. in a pint infufion, and directed two fpoonfuls to be given every two hours: this had the defired effect; the dropfy and the infanity difappeared together, and fhe had afterwards no other medicine but fome aperient pills to take occafionally.

C A S E XXXV.

April 12th. Mr. R——, Æt. 32. For the laft three or four years had had more or lefs of what was confidered as afthma;—it appeared to me Hydrothorax. I directed an infufion of Digitalis, which prefently removed his complaints. In *June* following he had a relapfe, and took two grains of the Pulv. fol. Digit. three times a day, which cured him after taking forty grains, and he has never had a return.

CASE

C A S E   XXXVI.

May 15th. Mrs. H——, Æt. 40. A spasmodic asthma, attended with symptoms of effusion. An infusion of Digitalis relieved her very considerably, and she lived four years afterwards without any relapse.

C A S E   XXXVII.

May 26th. R—— B——, Æt. 12. Scrophulous, consumptive, and at length anasarcous. Took Infus. Digital. without advantage. Died the *July* following.

C A S E   XXXVIII.

June 4th. Mrs. S——, of W——, Æt 49. Ascites and anasarca. Had taken many medicines; first from her apothecary, afterwards by the direction of a very judicious and very celebrated physician, but nothing retarded the increase of the dropsy. I first saw her along with the physician mentioned above, on the 14th of *May;* we directed an electuary of chrystals of tartar, and Seltzer water for common drink; this plan failing, as others had done before, we ordered the Infus. Digital. which in a few days nearly removed the dropsy. I then left her to the care of her physician; but her constitution was too much impaired to admit of restoration to health, and I understand she died a few weeks afterwards.

CASE

C A S E XXXIX.

June 13th. Mr. P———, Æt. 35. A very hard drinker, was attacked with a severe hæmoptoe, which was followed by afcites and anafarca. He had every appearance of difeafed vifcera, and his urine was fmall in quantity. The powder and the infufion of Digitalis were given at different times, but without the defired effect. Other medicines were tried, but in vain. Tapping prolonged his exiftence a few weeks, and he died early in the following autumn.

C A S E XL.

June 27th. Mr. W———, Æt. 37. An apparently afthmatic affection, gradually increafing for three or four years, which not yielding to the ufual remedies, he took the infufion of Digitalis. Two or three dofes made him very fick; but he thought his breathing relieved. After one week he took it again, and was fo much better as to want no other medicine.

In the courfe of the following winter he became hectic, and died confumptive about a year afterwards.

C A S E XLI.

July 6th. Mr. E———, Æt. 57. Hydrothorax and anafarca; his breath fo fhort that he could not
lie

lie down. After a trial of squill, fixed alkaly, and dulcified spirit of nitre, I directed Pulv. Digital. gr. 2, thrice a day. In four days he was able to come down stairs; in three days more no appearance of disease remained; and under the use of aromatics and small doses of opium, he soon recovered his strength.

C A S E XLII.

July 7th. Miss H—— of T——, Æt. 39. In the last stage of a phthisis pulmonalis became dropsical. She took the Digitalis without being relieved.

C A S E XLIII.

July 9th. Mrs. F————, Æt. 70. A chearful, strong, healthy woman; but for a few years back had experienced a degree of difficult breathing when in exercise. In the course of the last year her legs swelled, and she felt great fulness about her stomach. These symptoms continued increasing very fast, notwithstanding several attempts made by a very judicious apothecary to relieve her. The more regular practitioner failing, she had recourse to a quack, who I believe plied her very powerfully with Daphne laureola, or some drastic purge of that kind. I found her greatly reduced in strength, her belly and lower extremities swollen to an amazing size, her urine small in quantity, and her appetite greatly impaired. For the first fortnight of my attendance blisters were applied, solution of fixed alkaly, decoction of seneka with vitriolic æther,

chrystals

chryſtals of tartar, ſquill and cordial medicines were
ſucceſſively exhibited, but with no advantage. I
then directed Pulv. Fol. Digital. two grains every
four hours. After taking eighteen grains, the urine
began to increaſe. The medicine was then ſtopped.
The diſcharge of urine continued to increaſe, and
in five or ſix days the whole of the dropſical water
paſſed off, without any diſturbance to the ſtomach
or bowels. As the diſtenſion of the belly had been
very great, a ſwathe was applied, and drawn gradually tighter as the water was evacuated. As no pains
were ſpared to prevent the return of the dropſy,
and as the beſt means I could deviſe proved unequal
to my wiſhes, both in this and in ſome other caſes,
I ſhall take the liberty to point out the methods
I tried at different times in as conciſe a manner as
poſſible, for the knowledge of what will not do, may
ſometimes aſſiſt us to diſcover what will.

1780.

July 18th. Infuſum amarum, ſteel, Seltzer water.

September 22d. Neutral ſaline draughts, with tinct.
canthar.

26th. Pills of ſoap, garlic and millepedes.

30th. The ſame pills, with infuſum amarum.

October 11th. Pills of aloes, aſſafetida, and ſal martis, in the day-time, and mercury rubbed down,
at night.

December 21ſt. The accumulation of water now required a repetition of the Digitalis. It was directed in infuſion, a dram and half to eight ounces,
and an ounce and half given every fourth hour,
until

until its effects began to appear. The water was soon carried off.

30th. Sal diuretic. twice a day. To eat preserved garlic frequently.

1781.

February 1st. Pills of calomel, squill and gum ammoniac.

3d. Infusion of Digitalis repeated, and after the water was carried off, Dover's powder was tried as a sudorific.

March 18th Infuf Digital. repeated.

26th. Pills of sal martis and aromatic species, with infusum amarum.

May 5th. Being feverish; James's powder and saline draughts.

10th. Laudanum every night, and an opening tincture to obviate costiveness.

24th. Infuf. Digitalis, one ounce only every fourth hour, which soon procured a perfect evacuation of the water.

August 11th. Infuf. Digitalis.

October 19th. An emetic, and fol. Cicut. pulv. ten grains every six hours.

November 8th. A mercurial bolus at bed-time.

16th. Infuf. Digitalis.

December 23d. An emetic—Pills of seneka and gum ammoniac—Vitriolic acid in every thing she drinks.

25th. Squill united to small doses of opium.

1782.

January 2d. A troublesome cough—Syrup of garlic and oxymel of squills. A blister to the back.

4th. Tincture

4th. Tincture of cantharides and paregoric elixir.

28th. Infuf. Digitalis, half an ounce every morning, and one ounce every night, was now fufficient to empty her.

March 26th. Infuf. Digitalis; and when emptied,
vitriol of copper twice a day.

April 1ft. A cordial mixture for occafional ufe.

Two months afterwards a purging came on, which
every now and then returned, inducing great
weaknefs—her appetite failed, and fhe died in
in *July*.

INTERVALS.

From *July* 9th, 1780, to *December* 21ft, 171 days.
From *December* 21ft to *February* 3d, 1781, 34 days.
From *February* 3d to *March* 18th, 44 days.
From *March* 18th to *May* 24th, 66 days.
From *May* 24th to *Auguft* 11th, 79 days.
From *Auguft* 11th to *November* 16th, 98 days.
From *November* 16th to *January* 28th, 1782, 74
days.
From *January* 28th to *March* 26th, 57 days.

None of the accumulations of water were at all
equal to that which exifted when I firft faw her, for
finding fo eafy a mode of relief, fhe became impa-
tient under a fmall degree of preffure, and often
infifted upon taking her medicine fooner than I
thought it neceffary. After the 26th of *March* the
degree of effufion was inconfiderable, and at the
time of her death very trifling, being probably carried off by the diarrhœa.

CASE

C A S E XLIV

July 12th. Mr. H——, of A——, Æt. 60. In the laſt ſtage of a life hurried to a termination by free living, dropſical ſymptoms became the moſt diſtreſſing. He wiſhed to take the Digitalis. It was given, but afforded no relief.

C A S E XLV.

July 13th. Mr. S——, Æt. 49. Aſthma, or rather hydrothorax, anaſarca, and ſymptoms of a diſeaſed liver. He was directed to take two grains of Pulv. ſol. Digital. every two hours, until it produced ſome effect. It ſoon removed the dropſical and aſthmatic affections, and ſteel, with Seltzer water, reſtored him to health.

C A S E XLVI.

Auguſt 6th. Mr. L——, Æt. 35. Aſcites and anaſarca. Pulv. Digital. grains three, repeated every fourth hour, until he had taken two ſcruples, removed every appearance of dropſy in a few days. He was then directed to take ſolution of merc. ſublimat. and ſoon recovered his health and ſtrength.

C A S E XLVII.

Auguſt 16th. Mr. G——, of W——, Æt. 86. Aſthma of many years duration, and lately an incipient anaſarca, with a paucity of urine. He had never lived intemperately, was of a chearful diſpoſition, and very ſenſible: for ſome years back had

loſt

loft all relifh for animal food, and his only fupport
had been an ounce or two of bread and cheefe, or
a fmall flice of feed-cake, with three or four pints
of mild ale, in the twenty-four hours. After trying chryftals of tartar, fixed alkaly, fquills, &c. I
directed three grains of Pulv. fol. Digital. made
into pills, with G. ammoniac, to be given every fix
hours; this prefently occafioned copious difcharges
of urine, removed his fwellings, and reftored him
to his ufual ftandard of health.

C A S E XLVIII.

Auguft 17th. T—— B——, Efq. of K——,
Æt. 46. Jaundice, dropfy, and great hardnefs in
the region of the liver. Infufion of Digitalis carried off all the effufion, and afterwards a courfe of
deobftruent and tonic medicines removed his other
complaints.

C A S E XLIX.

Auguft 23d. Mr. C——, Æt. 58. (The perfon
mentioned at Cafe XXIII.) He had continued free
from dropfy until within the laft fix weeks; his appetite was now totally gone, his ftrength extremely
reduced, and the yellow of his jaundice changed to a
blackifh hue. The Digitalis was now tried in vain,
and he died fhortly afterwards.

C A S E L.

Auguft 24th. Mrs. W————, Æt. 39. Anafarcous legs and fymptoms of hydrothorax, confequent
to

to a tertian ague.   Three grains of Pulv. Digitalis,
given every fourth hour, occasioned a very copious
flow of urine, and she got well without any other
medicine.

C A S E LI.

August 28th.   Mr. J—— H——, Æt. 27.   In
consequence of very free living, had an ascites and
swelled legs.   I ordered him to take two grains of
Fol. Digital. pulv. every two hours, until it produced some effect; a few doses caused a plentiful
secretion of urine, but no sickness, or purging : in
six days the swellings disappeared, and he has since
remained in good health.

C A S E LII.

September 27th.   Mr. S——, Æt. 45.   Had been
long in an ill state of health, from what had been
supposed an irregular gout, was greatly emaciated,
had a sallow complexion, no appetite, costive bowels, quick and feeble pulse.   The cause of his complaints was involved in obscurity; but I suspected
the poison of lead, and was strengthened in this
suspicion, upon finding his wife had likewise ill
health, and, at times, severe attacks of colic; but
the answers to my enquiries seemed to prove my
suspicions fruitless, and, amongst other things, I
was told the pump was of wood. He had lately suffered extremely from difficult breathing, which I
thought owing to anasarcous lungs; there was also
a slight degree of pale swelling in his legs.   Pulv.
fol.

fol. Digital. made into pills, with gum ammoniac
and aromatic species, soon relieved his breathing.
Attempts were then made to assist him in other respects, but with little good effect, and some months
afterwards he died, with every appearance of a
worn out constitution.

About two years after this gentleman's death, I was
talking to a pump-maker, who, in the course of con-
versation, mentioned the corrosion of leaden pumps,
by some of the water in this town, and instanced
that at the house of Mr. S——, which he had replaced with a wooden one about three years before.
The lead, he said, was eaten away, so as to be very
thin in some places, and full of holes in others;—
this accidental information explained the mystery.

The deleterious effects of lead seem to be considerably modified by the constitution of the patient;
for in some families only one or two individuals
shall suffer from it, whilst the rest receive it with
impunity. In the spring of the year 1776, I was
desired to visit Mrs. H——,' of S—— Park, who
had repeatedly been attacked with painful colics,
and had suffered much from insuperable costiveness;
I suspected lead to be the cause of her complaints,
but was unable to trace by what means it was taken.
She was relieved by the usual methods; but, a few
months afterwards, I was desired to see her again:
her sufferings were the same as before, and notwithstanding every precaution to guard against costiveness, she was never in perfect health, and seldom
escaped

escaped severe attacks twice or thrice in a year; she had also frequent pains in her joints. I could not find any traces of similar complaints either in Mr. H——, the children, or the servants Mrs. H—— was a water drinker, and seldom tasted any fermented liquor. The pump was of wood, as I had been informed upon my first visit. Her health continued nearly in the same state for two or three years more, but she always found herself better if she left her own house for any length of time. At length it occurred to me, that though the pump was a wooden one, the piston might work in lead. I therefore ordered the pump rods to be drawn up, and upon examination with a magnifying glass, found the leather of the piston covered with an infinite number of very minute shining particles of lead. Perhaps in this instance the metal was so minutely divided by abrasion, as to be mechanically suspended in the water. The lady was directed to drink the water of a spring, and never to swallow that from the pump. The event confirmed my suspicions, for she gradually recovered a good state of health, lost the obstinate costiveness, and has never to this day had any attack of the colic.

C A S E LIII.

September 28th. Mrs. J——, Æt. 70. Ascites and very thick anasarcous legs and thighs, total loss of strength and appetite. Infusion of Digitalis was given, but, as had been prognosticated, with no good effect.

C A S E

C A S E LIV.

September 30th. Mr. A——, Æt. 57. A strong man; hydrothorax and swelled legs; in other respects not unhealthful. He was directed to take two grains of the Pulv. fol. Digit. made into a pill with gum ammoniac. Forty grains thus taken at intervals, effected a cure by increasing the quantity of urine, and he has had no relapse.

C A S E LV.

November 2d. Mr. P—— of T——, Æt. 42. A very strong man, drank a great quantity of strong ale, and was much exposed to alterations of heat and cold. About the end of summer found himself short winded, and lost his appetite. The dyspnœa gradually increased, he got a most distressing sense of tightness across his stomach, his urine was little, and high coloured, and his legs began to swell; his pulse slender and feeble. From the 20th of *September* I frequently saw him, and observed a gradual and regular increase of all his complaints, notwithstanding the use of the most powerful medicines I could prescribe. He took chrystals of tartar, seneka, gum ammoniac, saline draughts, emetics, tinct. of cantharides, spirits of nitre dulcified, squills in all forms, volatile alkaly, calomel, Dover's powder, &c. Blisters and drastic purgatives were tried, interposing salt of steel and gentian. I had all along felt a reluctance to prescribe the Digitalis in this case, from a persuasion that it would not succeed.

D   At

At length I was compelled to it, and directed one grain to be given every two hours until it should excite nausea. This it did; but, as I expected, it did no more. The reason of this belief will be mentioned hereafter. Five days after this last trial I gave him assafetida in large quantity, flattered by a hope that his extreme sufferings from the state of his respiration, might perhaps arise in part from spasm, but my hopes were in vain. I now thought of using an infusion of tobacco, and prescribed the following:

R. Fol. Nicotian. incif. ʒii.
 Aq. bull. ℔ſs.
 Sp. Vini rectif. ʒi digere per horam.

I directed a spoonful of this to be given every two hours until it should vomit. This medicine had no better effect than the former ones, and he died some days afterwards.

C A S E LVI.

November 6th. Mr. H——, Æt. 47. In the last stage of a phthisis pulmonalis, suffered much from dyspnœa, and anasarca. Squill medicines gave no relief. Digitalis in pills, with gum ammon. purged him, but opium being added, that effect ceased, and he continued to be relieved by them as long as he lived.

C A S E

C A S E LVII.

November 16th. Mrs. F———, Æt. 53. In *August* laſt was ſuddenly ſeized with epileptic fits, which continued to recur at uncertain intervals. Her belly had long been larger than natural, but without any perceptible fluctuation. Her legs and thighs ſwelled very conſiderably the beginning of this month, and now there was evidently water in the abdomen. The medicines hitherto in vain directed againſt the epileptic attacks, were now ſuſpended; and two grains of the Pulv. ſol. Digital. directed to be taken every ſix hours. The effects were moſt favourable, and the dropſical ſymptoms were ſoon removed by copious urinary diſcharges.

The attacks of epilepſy ceaſed ſoon afterwards. In *February*, 1781, there was ſome return of the ſwellings, which were ſoon removed, and ſhe now enjoys very good health. Does not the narrative of this caſe throw light upon the nature of the epilepſy which ſometimes attacks women, ſoon after the ceſſation of the menſtrual flux?

1781.

C A S E LVIII.

January 1ſt. Mrs. G———, of H———, Æt. 62. Aſcites and very large hard legs. After trying various medicines, under the direction of a very able phyſician, I ordered her to take one grain of Pulv.

Digital.

Digital. every six hours, but it produced no effect. Other Medicines were then tried to as little purpose. About the end of *February*, I directed an infusion of the Fol. Digital. but with no better success. Other methods were thought of, but none pioved efficacious, and she died a few weeks afterwards.

C A S E LIX.

January 3d. Mrs. B———, Æt. 53. Ascites, anasarca, and jaundice. After a purge of calomel and jallap, was ordered the Infusion of Digitalis: it acted kindly as a diuretic, and greatly reduced her swellings. Other medicines were then administered, with a view to her other complaints, but to no purpose, and she died about a month afterwards.

C A S E LX.

January 14th. Mr. B———, of D———. Jaundice and ascites, the consequences of great intemperance. Extremely emaciated; his tongue and sauces covered with apthous crusts, and his appetite gone. He first took tincture of cantharides with infusum amarum. then vitriolic salts, and various other medicines without relief; Infusum Digitalis was given afterwards, but was equally unsuccessful.

C A S E LXI.

February 2d. I was desired by the late learned and ingenious Dr. Groome. to visit Miss S———, a
young

young lady in the laſt ſtate of emaciation from a
dropſy. Every probable means to relieve her had
been attempted by Dr. Groome, but to no purpoſe; and ſhe had undergone the operation of the
paracenteſis repeatedly. The Doctor knew, he ſaid,
that I had cured many caſes of dropſy, by the Digitalis, after other more uſual methods had been
attempted without ſuccefs, and he wiſhed this lady
to try that medicine under my direction; after examining the patient, and enquiring into the hiſtory
of the diſeaſe, I was ſatisfied that the dropſy was
encyſted, and that no medicine could avail. The
Digitalis, however, was directed, and ſhe took it,
but without advantage. She had determined not to
be tapped again, and neither perſuaſion, nor diſtreſs
from the diſtenſion, could prevail upon her: I at length
propoſed to make an opening into the ſac, by means of
a cauſtic, which was done under the judicious management of Mr. Wainwright, ſurgeon, at Dudley.
The water was evacuated without any accident, and
the patient afterwards let it out herſelf from time to
time as the preſſure of it became troubleſome, until ſhe died at length perfectly exhauſted.

Query. Is there not a probability that this method, aſſiſted by bandage, might be uſed ſo as to
effect a cure, in the earlier ſtages of ovarium dropſy?

C A S E LXII.

February 27th. Mrs. O——, of T——, Æt. 52,
with a conſtitution worn out by various complicated
diſorders

diforders, at length became dropfical. The Digitalis was given in fmall dofes, in hopes of temporary
benefit, and it did not fail to fulfil our expectations.

C A S E LXIII.

March 16th. Mrs. P——, Æt. 47. Great debility, pale countenance, lofs of appetite, legs fwelled,
urine in fmall quantity. A dram of Fol. ficcat. Digital. in a half pint infufion was ordered, and an
ounce of this infufion directed to be taken every
morning. Myrrh and fteel were given at intervals.
Her urine foon increafed, and the fymptoms of
dropfy difappeared.

C A S E LXIV.

March 18th. Mr. W———, in the laft ftage
of a pulmonary confumption became dropfical. The
Digitalis was given, but without any good effect.

C A S E LXV.

April 6th. Mr. B———, Æt. 63. For fome
years back had complained of being afthmatical,
and was not without fufpicion of difeafed vifcera. The laft winter he had been moftly confined
to his houfe; became dropfical, loft his appetite,
and his fkin and eyes turned yellow. By the ufe
of medicines of the deobftruent clafs he became lefs
difcoloured, and the hardnefs about his ftomach
feemed to yield; but the afcites and anafarcous
fymptoms increafed fo as to opprefs his breathing
exceed-

exceedingly. Alkaline falts, and other diuretics failing of their effects, I ordered him to take an infuf. of Digitalis. It operated fo powerfully that it became neceffary to fupport him with cordials and blifters, but it freed him from the dropfy, and his breath became quite eafy. He then took foap, rhubarb, tartar of vitriol, and fteel, and gradually attained a good ftate of health, which he ftill continues to enjoy.

C A S E LXVI.

April 8th. Mr. B——, Æt. 60. A corpulent man, with a ftone in his bladder, from which at times his fufferings are extreme. He had been affected with what was fuppofed to be an afthma, for feveral years by fits, but through the laft winter his breath had been much worfe than ufual; univerfal anafarca came on, and foon afterwards an afcites. Now his urine was fmall in quantity and much faturated, the dyfuria was more dreadful than ever; his breath would not allow him to lie in bed, nor would the dyfuria permit him to fleep; in this diftrefsful fituation, after having ufed other medicines to little purpofe, I directed an infufion of Digitalis to be given. When the quantity of urine became more plentiful, the pain from his ftone grew eafier; in a few days the dropfy and afthma difappeared, and he foon regained his ufual ftrength and health. Every year fince, there has been a tendency to a return of thefe complaints, but he has recourfe to the infufion, and immediately removes them.

CASE

C A S E LXVII.

April 24th. Mr. M——, of C——, Æt. 57. Asthma, anasarca, jaundice, and great hardness and straitness across the region of the stomach. After a free exhibition of neutral draughts, alkaline salt, &c. the dropsy and difficult breathing remaining the same, he took Infusum Digitalis, which removed those complaints. He never lost the hardness about his stomach, but enjoyed very tolerable health for three years afterwards, without any return of the dropsy.

C A S E LXVIII.

April 25th. Mrs. J——, Æt. 42. Phthisis pulmonalis and anasarcous legs and thighs. She took the Infusum Digitalis without effect. Myrrh and steel, with fixed alkaly, were then ordered, but to no purpose.

C A S E LXIX.

May 1st. Master W——, of St——, Æt. 6. I found him with every symptom of hydrocephalus internus. As it was yet early in the disease, in consequence of ideas which will be mentioned hereafter, I directed six ounces of blood to be immediately taken from the arm; the temporal artery to be opened the succeeding day; the head to be shaven, and six pints of cold water to be poured upon it every fourth hour, and two scruples of strong mercuria curial ointment to be rubbed into the legs every day. Five days afterwards, finding the febrile symptoms very much abated, and judging the remaining disease to be the effect of effusion, I directed a scruple of Fol. Digital. siccat. to be infused in three ounces of water, and a table spoonful of the infusion to be given every third or fourth hour, until its action should be someway sensible. The effect was, an increased secretion of urine; and the patient soon recovered.

C A S E LXX.

May 3d. Mrs. B——, Æt. 59. Ascites and anasarca, with strong symptoms of diseased viscera. Infusum Digitalis was at first prescribed, and presently removed the dropsy. She was then put upon saline draughts and calomel. After some time she became feverish: the fever proved intermittent, and was cured by the bark.

C A S E LXXI.

May 3d. Mr. S——, Æt. 48. A strong man, who had lived intemperately. For some time past his breath had been very short, his legs swollen towards evening, and his urine small in quantity. Eight ounces of the Insuf. Digitalis caused a considerable flow of urine; his complaints gradually vanished, and did not return.

CASE

C A S E LXXII.

May 24th. Jofeph B——, Æt. 50. Afcites, ana-farca, and jaundice, from intemperate living. Infu-fion of Digitalis produced naufea, and lowered the frequency of the pulfe; but had no other fenfible ef-fects. His diforder continued to increafe, and killed him about two months afterwards.

C A S E LXXIII.

June 29th. Mr. B——, Æt. 60. A hard drinker; afflicted with afthma, jaundice, and dropfy. His appetite gone; his water foul and in fmall quantity. Neutral faline mixture, chryftals of tartar, vinum chalybeat. and other medicines had been prefcribed to little advantage. Infufion of Fol. Digitalis acted powerfully as a diuretic, and removed the moft ur-gent of his complaints, viz. the dropfical and afth-matical fymptoms.

The following winter his breathing grew bad again, his appetite totally failed, and he died, but without any return of the afcites.

C A S E LXXIV.

June 29th. Mr. A——, Æt. 58. Kept a public houfe and drank very hard. He had fymptoms of difeafed vifcera, jaundice, afcites, and anafarca. Af-ter taking various deobftruents and diuretics, to no purpofe, he was ordered the Infufion of Digitalis:
a few

a few dofes occafioned a plentiful flow of urine, relieved his breath, and reduced his fwellings; but,
on account of his great weaknefs, it was judged imprudent to urge the medicine to the entire evacuation of the water. He was fo much relieved as to
be able to come down ftairs and to walk about, but
his want of appetite and jaundice continuing, and
his debility increafing, he died in about two
months.

C A S E LXXV.

July 18th. Mrs. B——, Æt. 46. A little woman, and very much deformed. Afthmatical for
many years. For feveral months paft had been worfe
than ufual; appetite totally gone, legs fwollen,
fenfe of great fulnefs about her ftomach, countenance fallen, lips livid, could not lie down.

The ufual modes of practice failing, the Digitalis
was tried, but with no better fuccefs, and in about a
month fhe died; not without fufpicion of her death
having been accelerated a few days, by her taking
half a grain of opium. This may be a caution to
young practitioners to be careful how they venture
upon even fmall dofes of opium in fuch conftitutions, however much they may be urged by the patient to prefcribe fomething that may procure a little
reft and eafe.

CASE

C A S E   LXXVI.

August 12th. Mr. L——, Æt. 65, the person whose Case is recorded at No. XXIV, had a return of his infanity, after near two years perfect health. He was extremely reduced when I saw him, and the medicine which cured him before was now adminiftered without effect, for his weakness was fuch that I did not dare to urge it.

C A S E   LXXVII.

September 10th. Mr. V——, of S——, Æt. 47. A man of ftrong fibre, and the remains of a florid complexion. His difeafe an afcites and fwelled legs, the confeqnence of a very free courfe of life; he had been once tapped, and taken much medicine before I faw him. The Digitalis was now directed: it lowered his pulfe, but did not prove diuretic. He returned home, and foon after was tapped again, but furvived the operation only a few hours.

C A S E   LXXVIII.

September 25th. Mr. O——, of M——, Æt. 63. Very painful and general fwellings in all his limbs, which had confined him moftly to his bed fince the preceding winter; the fwellings were uniform, tenfe, and refifting, but the fkin not difcoloured. After trying guiacum and Dover's powder without advantage, I directed Infufion of Digitalis. It acted on the kidneys, but did not relieve him. It is not

easy

eafy to fay what the difeafe was, and the patient living at a diftance, I never learnt the future progrefs or termination of it.

C A S E LXXIX.

September 26th. Mr. D——, Æt. 42, a very fenfible and judicious furgeon at B——, in Staffordfhire, laboured under afcites and very large anafarcous legs, together with indubitable fymptoms of difeafed vifcera. Having tried the ufual diuretics to no purpofe, I directed a fcruple of Fol. Digital ficcat. in a four ounce infufion, a table fpoonful to be taken twice a day. The fecond bottle wholly removed his dropfy, which never returned.

C A S E LXXX.

September 27th. Mrs. E——, Æt. 42. A fat fedentary woman; after a long illnefs, very indiftinctly marked; had fymptoms of enlarged liver and dropfy. In this cafe I was happy in the affiftance of Dr. Afh. Digitalis was once exhibited in fmall dofes, but to no better purpofe than many other medicines. She fuffered great pain in the abdomen for feveral weeks, and after her death, the liver, fpleen, and kidneys were found of a pale colour, and very greatly enlarged, but the quantity of effufed fluid in the cavity was not more than a pint.

CASE

C A S E LXXXI.

October 28th. Mr. B——, Æt. 33. Had drank an immenſe quantity of mild ale, and was now become dropſical. He was a luſty man, of a pale complexion: his belly large, and his legs and thighs ſwollen to an enormous ſize. I directed the Infuſion of Digitalis, which in ten days completely emptied him. He was then put upon the uſe of ſteel and bitters, and directed to live temperately, which I believe he did, for I ſaw him two years afterwards in perfect health.

C A S E LXXXII.

November 14th. Mr. W——, of T——, Æt. 49. A luſty man, with an aſthma and anaſarca. He had taken ſeveral medicines by the direction of a very judicious apothecary, but not getting relief as he had been accuſtomed to do in former years, he came under my direction. For the ſpace of a month I tried to relieve him by fixed alkaly, ſeneka, Dovers powder, gum ammoniac, ſquill, &c. but without effect. I then directed Infuſion of Digitalis, which ſoon increaſed the flow of urine without exciting nauſea, and in a few days removed all his complaints.

CASE

1782.

C A S E LXXXIII.

January 23d. Mr. Q——, Æt. 74. A ſtone in his bladder for many years; dropſical for the laſt three months. Had taken at different times ſoap with ſquill and gum ammoniac; ſoap lees; chryſtals of tartar, oil of juniper, ſeneka, jallap, &c. but the dropſical ſymptoms ſtill increaſed, and the dyſuria from the ſtone became very urgent. I now directed a dram of the Fol. Digit. ſiccat. in a half pint infuſion, half an ounce to be given every ſix hours. This preſently relieved the dyſuria, and ſoon removed the dropſy, without any diſturbance to his ſyſtem.

C A S E LXXXIV.

January 27th. Mr. D——, Æt. 86. The debility of age and dropſical legs had long oppreſſed him. A few weeks before his death his breathing became very ſhort, he could not lie down in bed, and his urine was ſmall in quantity. A wine glaſs of a weak Infuſion of Digitalis, warmed with aromatics, was ordered to be taken twice a day. It afforded a temporary relief, but he did not long ſurvive.

C A S E LXXXV.

January 28th. Mr. D——, Æt. 35. A publican and a hard drinker. Aſcites, anaſarca, diſeaſed
viſcera

viscera, and slight attacks of hæmoptoe. A dram of Fol. Digital. sicc. in a half pint infusion, of which one ounce was given night and morning, proved diuretic and removed his dropsy. He then took medicines calculated to relieve his other complaints. The dropsy did not return during my attendance upon him, which was three or four weeks. A quack then undertook to cure him with blue vitriol vomits, but as I am informed, he presently sunk under that rough treatment.

C A S E   LXXXVI.

January 29th. Mrs. O——, of D——, Æt. 53. A constant and distressing palpitation of her heart, with great debility. From a degree of anasarca in her legs I was led to suspect effusion in the Pericardium, and therefore directed Digitalis, but it produced no benefit. She then took various other medicines with the same want of success, and about ten months afterwards died suddenly.

C A S E   LXXXVII.

January 31st. Mr. T——, of A——, Æt. 81. Great difficulty of breathing, so that he had not lain in bed for the last six weeks, and some swelling in his legs. These complaints were subsequent to a very severe cold, and he had still a troublesome cough. He told me that at his age he did not look for a cure, but should be glad of relief, if it could be obtained without taking much medicine. I directed an Infusion of Digitalis, a dram to eight ounces,

one

one spoonful to be taken every morning, and two at night. He only took this quantity; for in four days he could lie down, and foon afterwards quitted his chamber. In a month he had a return of his complaints, and was relieved as before.

C A S E LXXXVIII.

January 31ft. Mrs. J——, of S——, Æt. 67. A lufty woman, of a florid complexion, large belly, and very thick legs. She had been kept alive for fome years by the difcharge from ulcers in her legs; but the fores now put on a very difagreeable livid appearance, her belly grew ftill larger, her breath fhort, her pulfe feeble, and fhe could not take nourifhment. Several medicines having been given in vain, the Digitalis was tried, but with no better effect; and in about a month fhe died.

C A S E LXXXIX.

February 2d. Mr. B——, Æt. 73. An univerfal dropfy. He took various medicines, and Digitalis in fmall dofes, but without any good effect.

C A S E XC.

February 24th. Mafter M——, of W——, Æt. 10. An epilepfy of fome years continuance, which had never been interrupted by any of the various methods tried for his relief. The Digitalis was given for a few days, but as he lived at a diftance, fo that I could not attend to its effects, he only took one

E half

half pint infusion, which made no alteration in his
complaint.

C A S E   XCI.

March 6th. Mr. H——, Æt. 62. A very hard
drinker, and had twice had attacks of apoplexy. He
had now an afcites, was anafarcous, and had every
appearance of a difeafed liver. Small dofes of calomel, Dover's powder, infufum amarum, and fal
fodæ palliated his fymptoms for a while; thefe failing; blifters, fquills, and cordials were given without effect. A weak Infufion of Digitalis, well aro-
matifed, was then directed to be given in fmall
dofes. It rather feemed to check than to increafe
the fecretion of urine, and foon produced ficknefs.
Failing in its ufual effect, the medicine was no longer
continued; but every thing that was tried proved
equally inefficacious, and he did not long furvive.

C A S E   XCII.

May 10th. Mrs. P——, Æt. 40. Spafmodic afthma of many years continuance, which had frequently been relieved by ammoniacum, fquills, &c. but
thefe now failing in their wonted effects, an Infuf.
of Fol. Digitalis was tried, but it feemed rather to
increafe than relieve her fymptoms.

C A S E   XCIII.

May 22d. Mr. O——, of B——, Æt. 61. A
very large man, and a free liver; after an attack of
hemi-

hemiplegia early in the spring, from which he only partially recovered, became dropsical. The dropsy occupied both legs and thighs, and the arm of the affected side. I directed an Infusion of Digitalis in small doses, so as not to affect his stomach. The swellings gradually subsided, and in the course of the summer he recovered perfectly from the palsy.

C A S E XCIV.

July 5th. Mr. C——, of W——, Æt. 28. Had drank very freely both of ale and spirits; and in consequence had an ascites, very large legs, and great fulness about the stomach. He was ordered to take the Infusion of Digitalis night and morning for a few days, and then to keep his bowels open with chrystals of tartar. The first half pint of infusion relieved him greatly; after an interval of a fortnight it was repeated, and he got well without any other medicine, only continuing the chrystals of tartar occasionally. I forgot to mention that this gentleman, before I saw him, had been for two months under the care of a very celebrated physician, by whose direction he had taken mercurials, bitters, squills, alkaline salts, and other things, but without much advantage.

C A S E XCV.

March 6th. Mrs. W————, Æt. 36. In the last stage of a pulmonary consumption, took the Infus. Digitalis, but without any advantage.

C A S E   XCVI.

August 20th. Mr. P——, Æt. 43. In the year 1781 he had a severe peripneumony, from which he recovered with difficulty. At the date of this, when he first consulted me, the symptoms of hydrothoiax were pretty obvious. I directed a purge, and then the Infusum Digitalis, three drams to half a pint, one ounce to be taken every four hours. It made him sick, and occasioned a copious discharge of urine. His complaints immediately vanished and he remains in perfect health.

C A S E   XCVII.

September 24th. Mrs. R——, of B——, Æt. 35, the mother of many children. After her last lying in, three months ago, had that kind of swelling in one of her legs which is mentioned at No. VIII. XXVI, and XXXI. A considerable degree of swelling still remained; the limb was heavy to her feeling, and not devoid of pain. I directed a bolus of five grains of Pulv. Digitalis, and twenty-five of crude quicksilver rubbed down, with conserve of cynosbat. to be taken at bed-time, and afterwards an Infusion of red bark and Fol. Digitalis to be taken twice a day. There was half an ounce of bark and half a dram of the leaves in a pint infusion: the dose two ounces.

The leg soon began to mend, and two pints of the infusion finished the cure.

CASE

C A S E   XCVIII.

September 25th. Mr. R————, Æt. 60. Complained to me of a ficknefs after eating, and for
fome weeks paft he had thrown up all his food, foon
after he had fwallowed it.   He had taken various
medicines, but found benefit from none, and had
tried various kinds of diet.   He was now very thin
and weak; but had a good appetite.   As feveral
very probable methods had been prefcribed, and as
the ufual fymptoms of organic difeafe were abfent,
I determined to give him a fpoonful of the Infufion
of Digitalis twice a day; made by digefting two
drams of the dried leaves in half a pint of cinnamon
water.   From the time he began to take this medicine he fuffered no return of his complaint, and
foon recovered his flefh and his ftrength.

It fhould be obferved, that I had frequently feen
the Digitalis remove ficknefs, though prefcribed for
very different complaints.

C A S E   XCIX.

September 30th. Mrs. A————, Æt. 38. Hydrothorax and anafarca.   Her cheft was very confiderably deformed.   One half pint of the Digitalis Infufion entirely cured her.

C A S E C.

September 30th. Mr. R——, of W——, Æt. 47.
Hydrothorax and anasarca. An Infusion of Digitalis was directed, and after the expected effects from
that should take place, sixty drops of tincture of
cantharides twice a day. As he was costive, pills
of aloes and steel were ordered to be taken occasionally.

This plan succeeded perfectly. About a month
afterwards he had some rheumatic affections, which
were removed by guiacum.

C A S E CI.

October 2d. Mrs. R———, Æt. 60. Diseased
viscera; ascites and anasarca. Had taken various
deobstruent and diuretic medicines to little purpose.
The Digitalis brought on a nausea and languor, but
had no effect on the kidneys.

C A S E CII.

. *October* 12th. Mr. R——, Æt. 41. A publican,
and a hard drinker. His legs and belly greatly
swollen; appetite gone, countenance yellow, breath
very short, and cough troublesome. After a vomit
I gave him calomel, saline draughts, steel and bitters, &c. He had taken the more usual diuretics
before I saw him. As the dropsical symptoms increased, I changed his medicines for pills made of
soap

foap, containing two grains of Pulv. fol. Digital. in
each dofe, and, as he was coftive, two grains of
jallap. He took them twice a day, and in a week
was free from every appearance of dropfy. The
jaundice foon afterwards vanifhed, and tonics reftored him to perfect health.

C A S E   CIII.

October 12th. Mr. B——, Æt. 39. Kept a public houfe, drank very freely, and became dropfical;
he complained alfo of rheumatic pains. I directed
Infufion of Digitalis, half an ounce twice a day.
In eight days the fwellings in his legs and the fulnefs about his ftomach difappeared. His rheumatic
affections were cured by the ufual methods.

C A S E   CIV.

October 22d. Mafter B——, Æt. 3. Afcites and
univerfal anafarca. Half a grain of Fol. Digital.
ficcat. given every fix hours, produced no effect;
probably the medicine was wafted in giving. An
infufion of the dried leaf was then tried, a dram to
four ounces, two tea fpoonfuls for a dofe; this foon
increafed the flow of urine to a very great degree,
and he got perfectly well.

C A S E   CV.

October 30th. Mr. G——, of W——, Æt. 88.
The gentleman mentioned in No. XLVII. His
complaints and manner of living the fame as there
mentioned.

mentioned. I ordered an Infufion of the Digitalis, a dram and half to half a pint; one ounce to be taken twice a day; which cured him in a fhort time.

On *March* the 23d, 1784, he fent for me again. His complaints were the fame, but he was much more feeble. On this account I directed a dram of the Fol. Digitalis to be infufed for a night in four ounces of fpirituous cinnamon water, a fpoonful to be taken every night. This had not a fufficient effect; therefore, on the 22d of *April*, I ordered the infufion prefcribed two years before, which foon removed his complaints.—

He died foon afterwards, fairly worn out, in his ninetieth year.

C A S E   CVI.

November 2d. Mr. S———, of B——h——, Æt. 61. Hydrothorax and fwelled legs. Squills were given for a week in very full dofes, and other modes of relief attempted; but his breathing became fo bad, his countenance fo livid, his pulfe fo feeble, and his extremities fo cold, that I was apprehenfive upon my fecond vifit that he had not twenty-four hours to live. In this fituation I gave him the Infufum Digitalis ftronger than ufual, viz. two drams to eight ounces. Finding himfelf relieved by this, he continued to take it, contrary to the directions given, after the diuretic effects had appeared.

The

The ficknefs which followed was truly alarming; it continued at intervals for many days, his pulfe funk down to forty in a minute, every object appeared green to his eyes, and between the exertions of reaching he lay in a ftate approaching to fyncope. The ftrongeft cordials, volatiles, and repeated blifters barely fupported him. At length, however, he did begin to emerge out of the extreme danger into which his folly had plunged him; and by generous living and tonics, in about two months he came to enjoy a perfect ftate of health.

C A S E   CVII.

November 19th. Mafter S————, Æt. 8. Afcites and anafarca. A dram of Fol. Digitalis in a fix ounce infufion, given in dofes of a fpoonful, effected a perfect cure, without producing naufea.

1783.

The reader will perhaps remark, that from the middle of *January* to the firft of *May*, not a fingle cafe occurs, and that the amount of cafes is likewife lefs than in the preceding or enfuing years; to prevent erroneous conjectures or conclufions, it may be expedient to mention, that the ill ftate of my own health obliged me to retire from bufinefs for fome time in the fpring of the year, and that I did not perfectly recover until the following fummer.

CASE

C A S E CVIII.

January 15th. Mrs. G——, Æt. 57. A very fat woman; has been dropsical since *November* last; with symptoms of diseased viscera. Various remedies having been taken without effect, an Infusion of Digitalis was directed twice a day, with a view to palliate the more urgent symptoms. She took it four days without relief, and as her recovery seemed impossible it was urged no farther.

C A S E CIX.

May 1st. Mrs. D———, Æt. 72. A thin woman, with very large anasarcous legs and thighs; no appetite and general debility. After a month's trial of cordials and diuretics of different kinds, the surgeon who had scarified her legs apprehended they would mortify; she had very great pain in them, they were very red and black by places, and extremely tense. It was evident that unless the tension could be removed, gangrene must soon ensue. I therefore gave her Infusum Digitalis, which increased the secretion of urine by the following evening, so that the great tension began to abate, and together with it the pain and inflammation. She was so feeble that I dared not to urge the medicine further, but she occasionally took it at intervals until the time of her death, which happened a few weeks afterwards.

CASE

C A S E CX.

May 18th. I was defired to prefcribe for Mary Bowen, a poor girl at Hagley. Her difeafe appeared to me to be an ovarium dropfy. In other refpects fhe was in perfect health. I directed the Digitalis to be given, and gradually pufhed fo as to affect her very confiderably. It was done; but the patient ftill carries her big belly, and is otherwife very well.

C A S E CXI.

May 25th. Mr. G——, Æt. 28. In the laft ftage of a pulmonary confumption of the fcrophulous kind, took an Infufion of Digitalis, but without any advantage.

C A S E CXII.

May 31ft. Mr. H——, Æt. 27. In the laft ftage of a phthifis pulmonalis became dropfical. He took half a pint of the Infufum Digitalis in fix days, but without any fenfible effect.

C A S E CXIII.

June 3d. Mafter B————, of D——, Æt. 6. With an univerfal anafarca, had an extremely troublefome cough. An opiate was given to quiet the cough at night, and 2 tea fpoonfuls of Infuf. Digit. were ordered every fix hours. The dropfy was prefently removed; but the cough continued, his
flefh

flesh wasted, his strength failed, and some weeks afterwards he died tabid.

C A S E   CXIV.

June 19th. Mrs. L——, Æt. 28. A dropsy in the last stage of a phthisis. Infusum Digitalis was tried to no purpose.

C A S E   CXV.

June 20th. Mrs. H——, Æt. 46. A very fat, short woman; had suffered severely through the last winter and spring from what had been called asthma; but for some time past an universal anasarca prevailed, and she had not lain down for several weeks. After trying vitriolic acid, tincture of cantharides, squills, &c. without advantage, she took half a pint of Insuf. Digitalis in three days. In a week afterwards the dropsical symptoms disappeared, her breath became easy, her appetite returned, and she recovered perfect health. The infusion neither occasioned sickness nor purging.

C A S E   CXVI.

June 24th. Mrs. B——, Æt. 40. A puerperal fever, and swelled legs and thighs. The fever not yielding to the usual practice, I directed an Infusion of Fol. Digitalis. It proved diuretic; the swellings subsided, but the fever continued, and a few days afterwards a diarrhœa coming on, she died.

C A S E

C A S E CXVII.

July 22d. Mr. F——, Æt. 48. A strong man, of a florid complexion, in consequence of intemperance became dropsical, with symptoms of diseased viscera, great dyspnœa, a very troublesome cough, and total loss of appetite. He took mild mercurials, pills of soap, rhubarb, and tartar of vitriol, with soluble tartar and dulcified spirits of nitre in barley water. After a reasonable trial of this plan, he took squill every six hours, and a solution of assafœtida and gum ammoniac, to ease his breathing: finding no relief, I gave him chrystals of tartar with ginger; but his remaining health and strength daily declined, and he was not at all benefited by the medicines. I was averse to the use of Digitalis in this case, judging from what I had seen in similar instances of tense fibre, that it would not act as a diuretic. I therefore once more directed squill, with decoction of seneka and sal sodæ; but it was inefficacious. His strength being much broken down, I then ordered gum ammoniac, with small doses of opium, and infusum amarum, continuing the squill at intervals. At length I was urged to give the Digitalis, and considering the case as desperate, I agreed to do it. The event was as I expected; no increase in the urine took place; and the medicine being still continued, his pulse became slow, and he apparently sunk under its sedative effects. He was neither purged nor vomited; and had the Digitalis either been omitted

alto-

altogether, or fufpended upon its firft effects upon
the pulfe being obferved, he might perhaps have
exifted a week longer.

C A S E CXVIII.

July 26th. Mr. W——, of W——, Æt. 47.
Phthifis pulmonalis, jaundice, afcites, and fwelled
legs. As it was probable that the only relief I could
give in a cafe fo circumftanced, would be by carrying off the effufed fluids. I tried fquill and fixed
alkaly; and thefe failing, I ordered the Infufum
Digitalis. This had the defired effect, and, I believe, prolonged his life a few weeks.

C A S E CXIX.

Auguft 15th. Mrs. C———, Æt. 60. Afcites,
anafarca, difeafed vifcera, paucity of urine, and
total lofs of appetite. Thefe complaints had heretofore exifted repeatedly, and had been removed
by deobftruent and diuretic medicines; but in this
attack the fymptoms were fuffered to exift a longer
time and in a greater degree, before affiftance was
fought for. The remedies that ufed to relieve her
were now exhibited to no purpofe. Mild mercurials, foap, rhubarb, and fquill were tried; but fhe
grew rapidly worfe. Saline draughts with acetum
fcilliticum feemed for a few days to check the progrefs of her complaint, but they foon loft their effect, and diarrhœa enfued upon every attempt to
increafe the frequency of the dofe. Draughts with
Infuf. Digital. were then directed to be taken twice
a day.

a day. The effect was a powerful action on the kidneys, and a reduction of the swellings, but without sickness. A degree of appetite returned, but still the tendency to diarrhœa existed, and kept her weak. Tonic medicines were then tried, but without advantage, and in a month it was necessary to have recourse to the Digitalis again. It was directed in a half pint mixture; an ounce to be taken thrice in twenty-four hours. On the 2d day, finding her symptoms very much relieved, she took in the absence of her nurse, nearly a double dose of the medicine. The consequence was great sickness, languor continuing for several days, and almost a total stop to the secretion of urine, from the time the sickness commenced.

The case now became totally unmanageable in my hands, and, after a fortnight, I was dismissed, and another physician called in; but she did not long survive.

This was not the first, nor the last instance, in which I have seen too large a dose of the medicine, defeat the very purpose for which it was directed.

C A S E CXX.

August 22d. Mrs. S———, Æt. 36. Extreme faintness; anasarcous legs and thighs; great difficulty of breathing, troublesome cough, frequent chilly fits succeeded by hot ones; night sweats, and a tendency to diarrhœa. Apprehensive that the

more

more urgent symptoms were caused by water in the lungs, I directed an Infusion of Digitalis, with an ounce of diacodium to the half pint to prevent it purging, a wine glass full to be taken every night at bed-time, and a mixture with confect. cardiac. and pulv. ipecac. to be given in small doses after every loose stool.

On the fourth day she was better in all respects : had made a large quantity of water and did not purge. In a few days more she lost all her complaints, except the cough, which gradually left her, without any further assistance.

I was agreeably deceived in the event of this case, for I expected after the water was removed, to have had a phthisis to contend with.

C A S E   CXXI.

August 25th. T——W——, Esq; Æt, 50. A free liver, diseased viscera, belly very tense, and much swollen; fluctuation perceptible, but the swelling circumscribed; pulse 132. This gentleman was under the care of my very worthy friend Dr. Ash, who, having tried various modes of cure to no purpose, asked me if I thought the Digitalis would answer in this case. I replied that it would not, for I had never seen it effectual where the swelling appeared very tense and circumscribed. It was tried however, but did not lessen the swelling. I mention this case, to introduce the above remark, and also

to

to point out the great effect the Digitalis has upon the action of the heart; for the pulse came down to 96. He was afterwards tapped, and continued, for some time under our joint attendance, but the pulse never became quicker, nor did the swelling return.

C A S E   CXXII.

September 7th. Mr. L——, Æt. 43. After several severe attacks of ill formed gout, attended for some time past with jaundice and other symptoms of diseased viscera, the consequences of intemperate living, was sent to Buxton; from whence he returned in three weeks with ascites and anasarca. Under this complicated load of disease, I prescribed repeatedly without advantage, and at length gave him the Digitalis, which carried off the more obvious symptoms of dropsy; but the jaundice, loss of appetite, diseased viscera, &c. rendered his recovery impossible.

1784.

C A S E   CXXIII.

February 12th. Mrs. C——, Æt. 54. A strong short woman of a florid complexion; complained of great fulness across the region of the stomach; short breath, a troublesome cough, loss of appetite, paucity of urine; and had a brownish yellow tinge on her skin and in her eyes. She dated these complaints from a fall she had through a trap door about the beginning of winter. From the beginning of January to this time, she had been repeatedly let

F   blood

blood, had taken calomel purges with jallap; pills
of soap, rhubarb and calomel; saline julep with
acet. scillit. nitrous decoction, garlic, mercury rubbed
down, infus. amarum purg. &c. After the failure
of medicines so powerful, and seemingly so well
adapted, and during the use of which all the symptoms continued to increase, it was evident that a
favourable event could not be expected. However,
I tried the infusum Digitalis, but it did nothing. I
then gave her pills of quicksilver, soap and squill,
with decoction of dandelion, and after some time,
chrystals of tartar with ginger. Nothing succeeded
to our wishes, and the increase of orthopnœa compelled me occasionally to relieve her by drastic
purges, but these diminished her strength, more in
proportion than they relieved her symptoms. Tincture of cantharides, sal diureticus and various other
means were occasionally tried, but with very little
effect, and she died towards the end of March.

C A S E   CXXIV.

March 31st.   Miss W——, Æt. 60.   Had been
subject to peripneumonic affections in the winter.
She had now total loss of appetite, very great debility, difficult breathing; much cough, a considerable
degree of expectoration, and a paucity of urine. She
had been blooded, taken soap, assaf. and squill,
afterwards assaf. and ammon. with acet. scillit. :
but all her complaints increasing, a blister was applied to her back, and the Digitalis infusion directed
to be taken every night. The effect was an increased

secre-

secretion of urine, a considerable relief to her breath, and some return of appetite; but soon afterwards she became hectic, spat purulent matter, and died in a few weeks.

C A S E   CXXV.

April 12th. Mrs. H——, of L——, Æt. 61. In *December* last this Lady, then upon a visit in London, was attacked with severe symptoms of peripneumony. She was treated as an asthmatic patient, but finding no relief, she made an effort to return to her home to die. In her way through this place, the latter end of December, I was desired to see her. By repeated bleedings, blisters, and other usual methods, she was so far relieved, that she wished to remain under my care. After a while she began to spit matter and became hectic. With great difficulty she was kept alive during the discharge of the abscess, and about the end of March she had swelled legs, and unequivocal symptoms of dropsy in the chest. Other diuretics failing, on the 12th of April I was induced to give her the Digitalis in small doses. The relief was great and effectual. After an interval of fifteen days, some swellings still remaining in the legs, I repeated the medicine, and with such good effect. that she lost all her complaints, got a keen appetite, recovered her strength, and about the end of May undertook a journey of fifty miles to her own home, where she still remains in perfect health.

CASE

C A S E CXXVI.

April 17th. Mr. F——, Æt. 59. A very fat man, and a free liver; had long been subject to what was called asthma, particularly in the winter. For some weeks past his legs swelled, he had great sense of fullness across his stomach; a severe cough; total loss of appetite, thirst great, urine sparing, his breath so difficult that he had not lain down in bed for several nights. Calomel, gum ammoniac, tincture of cantharides, &c. having been given in vain, I ordered two grains of pulv. fol. Digitalis made into pills, with aromatic species and syrup, to be given every night. On the third day his urine was less turbid; on the fourth considerably increased in quantity, and in ten days more he was free from all complaints, and has since had no relapse.

C A S E CXXVII.

May 7th. Miss K——, Æt. 8. After a long continued ague, became hectic and dropsical. Her belly was very large, and she had a total loss of appetite. Half a grain of fol. Digital. pulv. with 2 gr. of merc. alcalis. were ordered night and morning, and an infusion of bark and rhubarb with steel wine to be given in the day time. Her belly began to subside in a few days, and she was soon restored to health. Two other children in the family, affected nearly in the same way, had died, from the parents being persuaded that an ague in the spring

was

was healthful and fhould not be ftopped.—I know
not how far the recovery in this cafe may be attributed to the Digitalis, but the child was fo near
dying that I dared not truft to any lefs efficacious
diuretic.

C A S E CXXVIII.

June 13th. Mr. C——, Æt. 45. A fat man, had
formerly drank hard, but not latterly : laft March
began to complain of difficult breathing, fwelled
legs, full belly, but without fluctuation, great thirft,
no appetite ; urine thick and foul ; complection
brownifh yellow. Mercurial medicines, diuretics
of different kinds, and bitters, had been trying for
the laft three months, but with little advantage. I
directed two grains of the fol. Digital. in powder to
be taken every night, and infuf. amar. with tinct.
facr. twice a day. In three days the quantity of his
urine increafed, in ten or twelve days all his fymptoms difappeared, and he has had no relapfe.

C A S E CXXIX.

June 17th. Mr. N——, of W——, Æt. 54.
A large man, of a pale complexion ; had been fubject to fevere fits of afthma for fome years, but now
worfe than ufual. The intermitting pulfe, the
great difturbance from change of pofture, and the
fwelled legs induced me to conclude that the exacerbation of his old complaint was occafioned by ferous
effufion. I directed pills with a grain and half of the

pulv.

pulv. Digital. to be taken every night, and as he was costive, jallap made a part of the composition. He was also directed to take mustardseed every morning and a solution of assafetida twice in the day. The effect of this plan was perfectly to our wishes, and in a short time he recovered his usual health. About half a year afterwards he died apoplectic.

C A S E CXXX.

Mary B——. A young unmarried woman. Her disease appeared to me a dropsy of the right ovarium. She took an infusion of Digitalis, but, as I expected with no good effect. She is still, I am informed, nearly in the same state.

C A S E CXXXI.

July 12th. Mrs. A——, of C——, Æt. 56. After a series of indispositions for several years, became dropsical ; and had long been confined to her chamber, unable to lie down or to walk. She was so feeble, her legs so much swelled, her breath so short, and the symptoms of diseased viscera so strong, that I dared not to entertain hopes of a cure ; but wishing to relieve her more urgent symptoms, directed quicksilver rubbed down and sol. Digital. pulv. to be made into pills : the dose, containing two grains of the latter, to be given night and morning. She was also ordered to take a draught with a dram of æther twice a day, and to have scapulary issues. Her breath was so much relieved, that

that she was able soon afterwards to come down stairs ; but her constitution was too much broken to admit of a recovery.

C A S E CXXXII.

July 16th. Mr. B——, of W——, Æt. 31. After a tertian ague of 12 months continuation, suffered great indisposition for 10 months more. He chiefly complained of great straitness and pain in the hypochondriac region, very short breath, swelled legs, want of appetite. He had been under the care of some very sensible practitioners, but his complaints increased, and he determined to come to Birmingham. I found him supported upright in his chair, by pillows, every attempt to lean back or stoop forward giving him the sensation of instantaneous suffocation. He said he had not been in bed for many weeks. His countenance was sunk and pale ; his lips livid ; his belly, thighs and legs very greatly swollen ; hands and feet cold, the nails almost black, pulse 160 tremulous beats in a minute, but the pulsation in the carotid arteries was such as to be visible to the eye, and to shake his head so that he could not hold it still. His thirst was very great, his urine small in quantity, and he was disposed to purge. I immediately ordered a spoonful of the infusum Digitalis every six hours, with a small quantity of laudanum, to prevent its running off by stool, and decoction of leontodon taraxacum to allay his thirst. The next day he began to make water freely, and could allow

allow of being put into bed, but was raised high
with pillows. Omit the infusion. That night he
parted with six quarts of water, and the next night
could lie down and slept comfortably. *July* 21st.
he took a mild mercurial bolus. On the 25th. the
diuretic effects of the Digitalis having nearly ceased,
he was ordered to take three grains of the pulv.
Digital. night and morning, for five days, and a
draught with half an ounce of vin. chalyb. twice a
day. *August* 15th. He took a purge of calomel and
jallap, and some swelling still remaining in his legs,
the Digitalis infusion was repeated. The water
having been thus entirely evacuated, he was ordered saline draughts with acetum scilliticum and
pills of salt of steel and extract of gentian. About
a month after this, he returned home perfectly well.

C A S E CXXXIII.

July 28th. Mr. A—— of W——, Æt. 29, became dropsical towards the close of a pulmonary
consumption. He was ordered 12 grains of pulv.
fol. cicutæ and 1 of Digitalis twice a day. No remarkable effect took place.

C A S E CXXXIV.

July 31. Mr. M——, Æt. 57. Hydrothorax.
A single grain of fol. Digital. pulv. taken every
night for three weeks cured him. The medicine
never made him sick, but increased his urine, which
became clear; whereas before it had been high coloured and turbid.

C A S E

C A S E CXXXV.

August 6th. Mr. C—— of E——, Æt. 42. Asthma and anasarca, the consequence of free living. He had been for some time under the care of an eminent physician of this place, but his complaints proving unusually obstinate, he consulted me. I directed an infusion of Digitalis to be taken every night, and a mixture with squill and tincture of cantharides twice every day. In about a week he became better, and continued daily mending. He has since enjoyed perfect health, having quitted a line of business which exposed him to drink too much.

C A S E CXXXVI.

August 6th. Mr. M—— of C——, Æt. 44. Ascites and anasarca, preceded by symptoms of the epileptic kind. He was ordered to take two grains of pulv. Digitalis every morning, and three every night; likewise a saline draught with syrup of squills, every day at noon. His complaints soon yielded to this treatment, but in the month of November following he relapsed, and again asked my advice. The Digitalis alone was now prescribed, which proved as efficacious as in the first trial. He then took bitters twice a day, and vitriolic acid night and morning, and now enjoys good health.

Before the Digitalis was prescribed, he had taken jallap purges, soluble tartar, salt of steel, vitriol of copper, &c.

C A S E

C A S E CXXXVII.

August 10th. Mrs. W——, Æt. 55. An ana-sarcous leg, and sciatica; full habit. After bleed-ing and a purge, a blister was applied in the man-ner recommended by Cotunnius; and two grains of sol. Digital. with fifteen of sol. cicutæ were di-rected to be taken night and morning. The medi-cine acted only as a diuretic; the pain and swelling of the limb gradually abated; and I have not heard of any return.

I must here bear witness to the efficacy of Co-tunnius's method of blistering in the sciatica, having used it in a great number of cases, and generally with success.

C A S E CXXXVIII.

August 16th. Mrs. A—— of S——, Æt. 78. About the middle of Summer began to complain of short breath, great debility, and loss of appetite. At this time there were evident marks of effusion in the thorax, and some swelling in the legs. The ad-vanced age, the weakness, and other circumstances of this patient, precluded every idea of her recovery: but something was to be attempted. Squills and other remedies had been tried; I therefore directed pills with two or three grains of the pulv. Digitalis to be taken every night for six nights, and a saline draught with forty drops of acetum scillit. twice in the day. She took but few of the draughts, seldom

more

more than half one at a time, for they purged her,
and she disliked them. The pills she took regularly,
and with the happiest effect, for she could lie down,
her breath was very much relieved, and a degree of
appetite returned. *Sept.* 4th, some return of her
symptoms demanded the further use of diuretics.
I was afraid to push the Digitalis in so hazardous a
subject, and therefore directed tinct. amara with tinct.
canthar. and pills of squill, seneka, salt of tartar and
gum ammoniac. These medicines did not at all
check the progress of the disease, and on the 26th
it became necessary to give the Digitalis again. The
pills were therefore repeated as before, and infus.
amarum with fixed alkaly ordered to be taken twice
a day. The event was as favorable as before ; and
from this time she had no considerable return of
dropsy, but languished under various nameless
symptoms, until the middle or end of November.

C A S E CXXXIX.

Aug. 16th. Mrs. P—— of S——, Æt. 50. For
a particular account of this patient, see Mr. Yonge's
second Case.

C A S E CXL.

Sept. 20th. B—— B——, Esq. A true spasmodic
asthma of many years continuance. After every
method of relief had failed; both under my management, and also under the direction of several of the
ablest physicians of this kingdom; I was induced to
give

give him an infusion of the Digitalis. It was continued until naufea came on, but procured no relief.

C A S E   CXLI.

October 5th.   Mr. R————, Æt. 43. *(The patient
mentioned at No.* 102.)   He had purfued his former
mode of life, and had now a return of his complaints, with evident marks of difeafed vifcera. His
belly not very large, but uncommonly tenfe. From
this circumftance I did not expect the Digitalis to
fucceed, and therefore tried for fome time to relieve him by the faline julep, with acet fcillitic.
jallap, mercury, fyrup of fquill, with aq. cinnam. decoction of Dandelion, &c.; but thefe being adminiftered without advantage, I was driven to the
Digitalis. As he was very weak and much emaciated, I only gave two grains night and morning for
five days. As no increafe of urine took place, I
ufed alkaline falt with tinct. cantharides :—This
proving equally unfuccefsful, on the 18th, I directed
two ounces of the infufum Digitalis night and morning. This was continued until naufea took place,
but the kidney fecretion was not increafed. Squill
with opium, deobftruents of different kinds, fubli-
mate folution, fixed alkaly, tobacco infufion, were
now fuccefsively tried, but with the fame want of
fuccefs. The fullnefs of his belly made it neceffary
to tap him, and by repeating this operation he
continued alive to the end of the year.

C A S E

C A S E CXLII.

October 19th. Mrs. R——, of B———, Æt. 47. Suppofed Afthma, of eighteen months duration. She had kept her room for four months, and could not lie down without great difturbance; was very thin, and had totally loft all inclination for food. She was directed to take two gr. of pulv. fol. Digital. night and morning for five days, and infufum amarum, at the hours of eleven and five. In the courfe of a week fhe was much relieved, and could remain in bed all night. After a few days interval fhe took the Digitalis for five days more, and was foon after that well enough to come down ftairs and conduct her family affairs.

In *April* 1785, fhe had a flight return, but not fuch as to confine her to her chamber. She experienced the fame relief from the fame medicine, but continuing it for feven days without interruption, it excited naufea.

C A S E CXLIII.

October 28th. Mr. A——, fubject to nephritis ealculofa: After an attack of that kind, had ftill a troublefome fenfe of weight about his loins, now and then rifing to pain, and a degree of dyfuria, together with a want of appetite. Thefe fymptoms not readily yielding to the ufual methods of treatment, I directed an infufion of Digitalis. The fourth dofe
caufed

caufed a copious flow of urine ; the fixth made him
fick, and he was more or lefs fick at times for three
days ; but felt no more of his complaints.

I don't believe it is at all neceffary to bring on
ficknefs in thefe cafes, but an unexpected abfence
from town prevented me from feeing him time
enough to ftop the exhibition of the medicine.

C A S E CXLIV.

October 31ft. Mrs. C——, of W——, Æt. 67.
Afthma, and very thick hard legs of long continuance. The laft month or two her breath worfe than
ufual, her belly fwollen, her thighs anafarcous, and
her urine in fmall quantity. After trying garlic,
fquill, and purgatives without advantage, I directed
the Digital. Infuf. After taking about five ounces,
her urine from thick and turbid, changed to clear
and amber coloured, its quantity confiderably increafed, and her breathing eafy. Contrary to my
orders, but impelled by the relief fhe had found,
fhe finifhed the remaining three ounces of the infufion, which made her very fick, and the free flow
of urine immediately ceafed. No medicine was
adminiftered for a fortnight, during which time her
complaints increafed. I then directed an infufion
of tobacco, which affected her head, but did not
increafe her urine. She had recourfe again to the
Digitalis infufion, which once more removed the
fulnefs of the belly, reduced the fwellings of her
thighs, and relieved her breath, but had no effect
upon her legs.

CASE

C A S E   CXLV.

Nov. 2d. Miſs B—— of C——, Æt. 22. A very evident fluctuation in the abdomen, which was conſiderably diſtended, whilſt the reſt of her frame was greatly emaciated. The preſence of cough, hectic fever, and other circumſtances, made it probable that this apparent aſcites was cauſed by a purulent, and not a watery effuſion. However it was poſſible I might be miſtaken ; the Digitalis was therefore given, but without any advantage.

The further progreſs of the diſeaſe confirmed my firſt opinion, and ſhe died conſumptive.

C A S E   CXLVI.

Nov. 4th. Mr. P—— of M——, Æt. 40. Subject to troubleſome nephritic complaints, and after the laſt attack did not recover, or void the gravelly concretions as uſual, a ſenſe of weight. acroſs his loins continuing very troubleſome. The uſual medicines failing to relieve him, I ordered four grains of puly. Digital. to be taken every other night for a week, and fifteen grains of mild fixed vegetable alkaly to be ſwallowed twice a day in barley water. He ſoon loſt all his complaints ; but we muſt not in this caſe too haſtily attribute the cure to the Digitalis, as the alkaly has alſo been found a very uſeful medicine in ſimilar diſorders.

CASE

C A S E   CXLVII.

Nov. 4th. Mr. B—— of N——, Æt. 60. Had been much subject to gout, but his constitution being at length unable to form regular fits, he became dropsical. Pulv. sol. Digital. in doses of two or three grains, at bed-time, gave him some relief, but did not perfectly empty him. About three months afterwards he had occasion to take it again; but it then produced no effect, and he was so debilitated that it was not urged further.

C A S E   CXLVIII.

Nov. 8th. Mr. G——, Æt. 35. In the last stage of a phthisis pulmonalis, was attacked with a most urgent and painful difficulty of breathing. Suspecting this distress might arise from watery effusion in the chest, I gave him Digitalis, which relieved him considerably; and during the remainder of his life his breath never became so bad again.

C A S E   CXLIX.

Nov. 13th. Mrs. A—— of W——h——, Æt. 68. One of those rare cases in which no urine is secreted. It proved as refractory as usual to remedies, and not having ever succeeded in the cure of this disease, I determined to try the Digitalis. It was given in infusion, and, after a few doses, the secretion of a small quantity of urine seemed to justify the attempt. The next day, however, the se-
cretion

cretion ceafed, nor could it be excited again, tho'
at laft the medicine was pufhed fo as to occafion
ficknefs, which continued at intervals for three
days.

C A S E CL.

Nov. 20th. Mrs. B——, Æt. 28. In the laft
ftage of a pulmonary confumption became dropfical. I directed three grains of the pulv. Digital. to
be taken daily, one in the morning, and two at
night. She took twenty grains without any fenfible effect.

C A S E CLI.

Nov. 23d. Mafter W——, Æt. 7. Suppofed
hydrocephalus internus. A grain of pulv. fol. Digitalis was directed night and morning. After
three days, no fenfible effects taking place, it was
omitted, and the mercurial plan of treatment
adopted. The child lived near five months afterwards. Upon diffection near four ounces of water
were found in the ventricles of the brain.

C A S E CLII.

Nov. 26th. Mrs. W——, Æt. 65. I had attended this lady laft winter in a very fevere peripneumony, from which fhe narrowly efcaped with
her life. When the cold feafon advanced this winter, fhe perceived a difficulty in breathing, which gradually became more and more troublefome. I found
her

her much harrasfed by a cough, which occasioned her to expectorate a little: the least motion increased her dyspnœa; she could not lie down in bed; her legs were considerably swelled, her urine small in quantity. I directed two grains of pulv. Digitalis made into a pill with gum ammoniac, to be taken every night, and to promote expectoration, a squill mixture twice in the day. Her urine in five days became clear and copious, and in a fortnight more she lost all her complaints, except a cough, for which she took the lac ammoniacum.

It is not improbable that the squill might have some share in this cure.

C A S E CLIII.

December 7th. Mr. H——, Æt. 42. A large fat man, very subject to gravelly complaints. After an attack in the usual manner, continued to feel numbness in his lower limbs, and a sense of weight across his loins. I directed infusum Digitalis to be given every six hours. Six ounces made him sick, and he took no more. The next day his urine increased, a good deal of sand passed with it, and he lost his disagreeable feels, but the sickness did not entirely cease before the fourth day from its commencement.

CASE

C A S E   CLIV.

December 27th.   Mr. B——, of H——, Æt. 55.
Symptoms of hydrothorax, at firſt obſcurely, afterwards more diſtinctly marked.   Many things were tried, but the ſquill alone gave relief.   At length this failed.   About the third month of the diſeaſe, a grain of pulv. Digital. was ordered to be taken night and morning.   This produced the happieſt effects.   In *March* following he had ſome ſlight ſymptoms of relapſe, which were ſoon removed by the ſame medicine, and he now enjoys good health. For a more particular narrative ſee caſe the firſt, communicated by Mr. Yonge.

C A S E   CLV.

December 31ſt.   Mrs. B——, of E——, Æt. 50.
An ovarium dropſy of long continuance.   She took three grains of pulv. Digital. every night at bed time, for a fortnight, but without any effect.

C A S E   CLVI.

A poor man in this town, after his kidneys had ceaſed to ſecrete urine for ſeveral days, was ſeized with hickup, fits of vomiting, and tranſient delirium. After examination I was ſatisfied the diſeaſe was the ſame as that mentioned at CXLIX.   A very experienced apothecary having tried various methods to relieve him, I deſpaired of any ſucceſs, but determined to try the Digitalis.   It was accordingly given

G 2

in

in infusion. At first it checked the vomitings, but did not occasion any secretion of urine.

1 7 8 5.

The cases which have occurred to me in the course of this year, are numerous ; but as the events of some of them are not yet sufficiently ascertained, I think it better to withhold them at present.

HOSPITAL

HOSPITAL CASES,

Under the Direction of the Author.

THE four following cases were drawn out at my request by Mr. Cha. Hinchley, late apothecary to the Birmingham Hospital. They are all the Hospital cases for which the Digitalis was prescribed by me, whilst he continued in that office.

CASE CLVII.

March 15th, 1780. John Butler, Æt. 30. Asthma and swelled legs. He was directed to take myrrh and steel every day, and three spoonfuls of infusum Digitalis every night. On the 8th of April he was discharged, cured of the swellings and something relieved of his asthmatic affections.

CASE CLVIII.

November 18th, 1780. Henry Warren, Æt. 60. This man had a general anasarca and ascites, and was moreover so asthmatic, that, neither being able to sit in a chair nor lie in bed, he was obliged constantly to walk about, or to lean forward against a window or table. You prescribed for him thus.

G 3 R. Aq.

R. Aq. cinn. spt. ℥iv.

 Oxymel. scillit.

 Syr. scillit. aa. ℥i. m. cap. cochlear. larg. sexta

 quaque horâ.

This medicine producing no increased discharge
of urine, on the 25th you ordered the infusion of
Digitalis, two spoonfuls every four hours. After
taking this for thirty six hours, his urine was discharged in very great quantity; his breath became
easy, and the swellings disappeared in a few days,
though he took no more of the medicine. On the
2d of *December* he was ordered myrrh and lac ammoniacum, which he continued until the 23d, when
he was discharged cured, and is now in good health.

C A S E   CLIX.

November 3d, 1781. Mary Crockett, Æt. 40.
Ascites and universal anasarca. For one week she
took sal. diureticus and tincture of cantharides, but
without advantage. On the 10th you directed the
infusion of Digitalis, a dram and half to half a pint,
an ounce to be taken every fourth hour. Before
this quantity was quite finished, the urine began to
be discharged very copiously. The medicine was
then stopped as you had directed. On the 15th,
being costive, she took a jallap purge, and on the
24th she was discharged cured.

C A S E   CLX.

March 16th, 1782. Mary Bird, Æt. 61. Great
fullness about the stomach; diseased liver, and ana-
           farcous

farcous legs and thighs. For the firſt week ſquill was tried in more forms than one, but without advantage. On the 22d ſhe began with the Digitalis, which preſently removed all the ſwelling.

She was then put upon the uſe of aperient medicines and tonics, and on the firſt of *Auguſt* was diſcharged perfectly cured.

––––––––––––

The three following Caſes were drawn up and communicated to me by Mr. Bayley, who ſucceeded Mr. Hinchley as apothecary to the Hoſpital at Birmingham:

DEAR SIR,   Shiffnal, April 26th, 1785.

DURING my reſidence in the Birmingham General Hoſpital, I had frequent opportunities of ſeeing the great effects of the Digitalis in dropſy. As the exhibition of it was in the following inſtances immediately under your own direction, I have drawn them up for your inſpection, previous to your publiſhing upon that excellent diuretic. Of its efficacy in dropſy I have conſiderable evidence in my poſſeſſion, but conſider myſelf not at liberty to ſend you any other caſes except thoſe you had yourſelf the conduct of. The Digitalis is a very valuable acquiſition to medicine; and, I truſt, it will ceaſe to be dreaded when it is well underſtood.

I am, Sir, your obedient,
And very humble ſervant,
W. BAYLEY.
CASE

C A S E   CLXI.

Mary Hollis, aged 62, was admitted an out patient of the Birmingham General Hofpital *February*
12th, 1784, labouring under all the effects of hydrothorax; her dread of fuffocation during fleep
was fo great, that fhe always repofed in an elbow
chair. She was directed to take two grains of Digitalis in powder every night and morning, and for
a few days found great relief; but, on the eighth
day, as fhe had complained of ficknefs, and had
been confiderably purged, fhe was ordered to defift
taking any more of her powders. On the 14th day
fhe was ordered an ounce of the following infufion
twice in a day: R. Fol. Digital. purp. ficc. 3ifs. aq.
bullient. ℔fs. digere per femi-horam, colaturæ adde
tinct. aromatic 3i. This infufion did not purge,
but fometimes excited naufea, though not fufficient
to prevent her from continuing its ufe. She grew
gradually better, and on the 6th of *May* was difcharged perfectly cured. The diuretic effects of the
Digitalis were in this inftance immediate.

C A S E   CLXII.

Edward James, Æt. 21. Admitted *March* 20th,
1784. Complained of great difficulty of breathing, pain in his head, and tightnefs about the ftomach, with a trifling fwelling of his legs. Ordered
pil. fcillit. 3i. ter de die. On the third day his legs
much more fwelled, his breathing more difficult,
and in every refpect worfe; his pulfe very fmall
and

and quick, complained when he turned in bed, of
fomething like water rolling from one fide of the
thorax to the other. A remarkable bluenefs about
the mouth and eyes, and purged confiderably from
the pil. fcill. Ordered to omit the pills and to
take ʒi. of infuf. Digitalis every eight hours; the
proportion ʒifs. to eight ounces of water and ʒi. of
aq. n. m. fp.—7th Day, The infufion had neither
purged, nor vomited him: he only complained once
or twice of giddinefs. His belly was now very hard,
rather black on the right fide the navel, and his legs
amazingly fwelled. Ordered a bolus with rhubarb
and calomel, to be taken in the morning, and ʒii.
julep falin. cum tinct. canthar. gutt. forty ter die.
—12th Day, nearly in the fame ftate, except his
breathing which was fomewhat more difficult, being
now obliged to have his head confiderably raifed.
Perfiftat—From this day to the 32d day he became
hourly worfe. His belly which at firft was only
hard, now evidently contained a large quantity of
water, his legs were more fwelled, and a large fpha-
celated fore appeared upon each outer ancle. Refpiration was fo much obftructed, that he was obliged
to fit quite upright to prevent fuffocation. He made
very little water, not more than eight ounces in a
day and a night, and was much emaciated. Ordered
his purging bolus again, and ʒii. of a mixture with
fal diuretic. ʒfs. to ʒxii. three times in a day, and
a poultice with ale grounds to his legs.

54th day. To this period there was not the leaft
probability of his exifting; his legs and thighs were
one

one continued blubber, his thorax quite flat, and
his belly fo large that it meafured within one inch
as much as a woman's in this Hofpital the day fhe.
was tapped, and from whom twenty feven pounds
of coagulable lymph were taken. He made about
three ounces of water in twenty-four hours: his
penis and fcrotum were aftonifhingly fwelled, and
no difcharge from the fores upon his legs. Ordered
to take a pill with two grains of powdered Fox-glove
night and morning. For a few days no fenfible
effect, but about the 60th day he complained of
being continually giddy, and had fome little pain
in his ftomach. He now made much more water,
and dared to fleep. His appetite which through the
whole of his illnefs had been very bad, was alfo better. 66th day. Breathing very much relieved, the
quantity of water he made was three chamber pots
full in a day and a night, each pot containing two
quarts and four ounces, moderately full. Ordered
to continue his pills, and his legs which were very
flabby, to be rolled.

69th day. His belly nearly reduced to its natural
fize, ftill made a prodigious quantity of water, his
appetite very good, habit of body rather lax, and
his complexion ruddy. On the 2d of *June*, being
ftill rather weak, he was ordered decoct. cort. ʒii.
ter de die ; and on the 12th was difcharged from
this Hofpital perfectly cured.

W. BAYLEY.

Mr,

Mr. Bayley's refpectful compliments to Doctor Withering: he fends the cafe of Edward James, which he believes is pretty correct. He laments not having it in his power to fend the meafure of his belly, having unfortunately miflaid the tape: he heard from James yefterday, and he is perfectly well.

General Hofpital, Auguft 5, 1784.

C A S E   CLXIII.

On the 26th *February*, 1785, Sarah Ford, aged 42, was admitted an out-patient of the Birmingham General Hofpital: fhe complained of confiderable pain in her cheft, and great difficulty of breathing, her face was much fwelled and her thighs and legs were anafarcous. She had extreme difficulty in making water, and with many painful efforts fhe did not void more than fix ounces in twenty-four hours. She had been in this fituation about fix weeks, during which time fhe had taken ammoniacum, olibanum, and large quantities of fquills, without any other effect than frequent ficknefs. Upon her commencing an Hofpital patient, the following medicine was exhibited. R. gum ammoniac ʒii. pulv. fol. Digital. purp. ɔ'i. fp. lavand. comp. ut fiat pil. 40. cap. ii. nocte maneque. She continued the ufe of thefe pills for a few days, without any fenfible effect. On the eighth day her breathing was much relieved, her legs and thighs were not fo much fwelled, and in a day and
a night

a night fhe made five pints of water.   By the 12th
day her legs and thighs were nearly reduced to their
natural fize.   She continued to make water in large
quantities, and had loft her pain in the thorax.   To
the 20th of *March*, fhe made rapid advances towards
health, when not a fymptom of difeafe remaining,
fhe was difcharged.

COMMU-

COMMUNICATIONS

FROM CORRESPONDENTS.

———————

London, Norfolk-street,
May 31st, 1785.

Sir,

I HAD the favour of your letter laſt week;
and I ſhall be very happy if I can give you any
intelligence relating to the Foxglove, that can anſwer the purpoſe in which you are ſo laudably engaged.

It is true that my brother, the late Dr. Cawley,
was greatly relieved, and his life, perhaps, prolonged for a year, by a decoction of the Foxglove
root; but why it had not a more laſting effect, it is
neceſſary I ſhould tell you that he had all the ſigns
of a diſtempered viſcera, long before any watery
ſwellings appeared; it was manifeſt that his dropſy
was merely ſymptomatic, and he could therefore only from time to time have any relief from medicine. In the year 1776, he returned from London to Oxon. having conſulted ſeveral phyſicians
at the former place, and Dr. Vivian at the latter,
but without any ſucceſs; and he was then told of
a carpenter at Oxon. that had been cured of a
Hydrops pectoris by the Foxglove root, and as he

was

was a younger, and in other refpect an healthy man, his cure, I believe, remains a perfect one.

I did not attend my brother whilst he took the medicine, and therefore I cannot fpeak precifely to the operation of it; but I remember, by his letters, that he was dreadfully fick and ill for feveral days before the fecretion of urine came on, but which it did do to a great degree; relieved his breath, and greatly leffened the fwelling in his legs and thighs; but the two inftances I have lately feen in this part of the world, are much ftronger proofs of the efficacy of it than my brother's cafe.

I am, &c.
ROBERT CAWLEY.

N. B. Whenever I have another opportunity of giving the Foxglove, it fhall be in fmall dofes:— In which I fhould hope it might fuceed, although it might be more flowly. If you fhould try it with fuccefs, I fhould be glad to know what mode you made ufe of.

Dr. Cawley's prefcription.

R. Rad. Digital. purpur. ficcat. et contuf. ʒii.
Coque ex aq. font. ℔ii. ad ℔i. colat. liquor. adde aq junip. comp. ʒii.
Mell. anglic ʒi. m. fumat cochl. iv. omni nocte h. f. et mane.

I have

—I have elfewhere remarked, that when the Digitalis has been properly given, and the diuretic effects produced, that an accidental over-dofe bringing on ficknefs, has flopped the fecretion of urine. In the prefent inftance it likewife appears, that violent ficknefs may be excited, and continue for feveral days without being accompanied by a flow of urine; and it is probable that the latter circumftance did not take place, until the feverity of the former abated. If Dr. Cawley had not had a conftitution very retentive of life, I think he muft have died from the enormous dofes he took; and he probably would have died previous to the augmentation of the urinary difcharge. For if the root from which his medicine was prepared, was gathered in its active ftate, he did not take at each dofe lefs than *twelve* times the quantity a ftrong man ought to have taken. Shall we wonder then that patients refufe to repeat fuch a medicine, and that practitioners tremble to prefcribe it? Were any of the active and powerful medicines in daily ufe to be given in dofes *twelve* times greater than they are, and thefe dofes to be repeated without atttention to the effects, would not the patients die, and the medicines be condemned as dangerous and deleterious?—Yet fuch has been the fate of Foxglove!

A Letter

A Letter to the Author, from Mr. BODEN, Surgeon, at Brofeley, in Shropfhire.

Dear Sir, Brofeley, 25th May, 1785.

HAVE inclofed the prefcriptions that contained the fol. Digital which I gave to Thomas Cooke and Thomas Roberts.

Thomas Cooke, Æt. 49, had been ill about two or three weeks. When I faw him he had no appetite, and a conftant thirft : a fullnefs and load in the ftomach : the thighs, legs and hands, much fwell'd, and the face and throat in a morning ; was coftive, and made but little water, which was high coloured ; the pulfe very weak, and his breath exceeding bad. *June* 17th. R. Argent. viv ʒi. conf. cynofbat. Əii. fol. Digital. pulv. gr. xv. f. pil. xxiv. capt. ii. omni nocte horâ decubitus. He was likewife purged by a bolus of argent. viv. jallap, Digit. elaterium and calomel, which was repeated on the fourth day, to the third time. From *June* 17th to the 29th, the fymptoms were moftly removed, making water freely, and having plenty of ftools ; in a week after he was perfectly well, and remains fo ever fince. The cure was finifhed by fteel and bitters.

Thomas Roberts, Æt. 40, had a deformed cheft, was obliged to be almoft in an erect pofture when in bed ; the other fymptoms were nearly the fame as Cooke's. *Auguft* 3d. The pills prefcribed *June* 17th

17th for Cooke.——17th. A purging bolus of jalap and Digitalis, once a week. He continued the medicines till the latter end of *Auguſt*, when he got very well; but the complaint returned in *Jan.* worſe than before. He is now much better, but I have great reaſon to believe the liver to be diſeaſed.

I am, with the greateſt reſpect,

Your very obliged humble ſervant,

DANIEL BODEN.

P. S. The ſecond patient, on his relapſe, took Digitalis again, combined with other things.

CASE communicated by Mr. CAUSER, Surgeon, at Stourbridge, Worceſterſhire.

Mr. P—— of H—— M——, in the pariſh of Kingſwinford, aged about 60; had been a ſtrong healthy, robuſt, corpulent man; worked hard early in life at edge-tool making, and drank freely of ſtrong malt liquor; for many years had been ſubject to gout in the extremities; for a few years paſt had been very aſthmatic, and the gout in the extremities gradually decreaſed. When I firſt ſaw him, which was *Sept.* 12, 1779, his legs were anaſarcous, his belly much ſwelled, and an evident fluctuation of water. His breathing very bad, an irregular pulſe, and unable to lie down. His eaſieſt

H   poſture

posture was standing with his body leaning over a chair, in which situation he would continue many hours together, labouring for breath, with the sweat trickling down his face very profusely; the urine in very small quantity. Diuretics of every kind I could think of were used with very little or no advantage. Blisters applied to the legs relieved very considerably for a time, but by no means could I increase the urinary discharge. Warm stomachic medicines were given, and at the same time sinapisms applied to the feet, in hopes of enticing gout to the extremities, but without any good effect.— *November* 22d. The swelling considerably increasing, an emetic of acet. scillitic. was given, which acted very violently, and increased the urinary discharge considerably. He continued better and worse, using different kinds of diuretic and expectorating medicines until *September* 1781, when the disease was so much worse, I did not expect he could live many days. The acet. scillitic. was repeated, a table spoonful every half hour, till it acted briskly upwards and downwards; but without increasing the urinary discharge.—On the 17th of *September* I infused ʒiii. of the fol. Digitalis in ʒvi. of boiling water, for four hours; then strained it, and added ʒi. of tinct. aromatica.—On the 18th he began by taking one spoonful, which he was to repeat every half hour, till it made him very sick, unless giddiness, loss of sight, or any other disagreeable effect took place. I had never given the medicine before, and had prepared him to expect the operation to be very severe. I saw him again on the 21st; he

had

had taken the medicine regularly, till the whole quantity was confumed, without perceiving the leaft effect of any kind from it, and continued well till the evening of the following day, when a little ficknefs took place, which increafed, but never fo as to occafion either vomiting or purging, but a furprifing difcharge of urine. The faliva increafed fo as to run out of his mouth, and a watery difcharge from his eyes; thefe difcharges continued, with a continual ficknefs, till the fwelling was totally gone, which happened in three or four days. He afterwards took fteel and bitters; and continued very comfortably, without any return of his dropfy, until the the 7th of *April* 1782, when he was feized with an epidemic cough, which was very frequent with us at that time. His fwellings now returned very rapidly, with the greateft difficulty in breathing, and he died in a few days. Blifters and expectorating medicines were ufed on this laft return.

Extract of a Letter from Mr. CAUSER.

Mrs. S——, the fubject of the following Cafe, was as ill as it is poffible for woman to be and recover; from the inefficacy of the medicines ufed, I am convinced no medicine would have faved her but the Digitalis. I never faw fo bad a cafe recovered; and it fhews, that in the moft reduced ftate of body, the medicine in fmall dofes, will prove fafe and efficacious.

N. B. The

N. B. The Digitalis, in pills, never occafioned the leaft ficknefs. She took two boxes of them.

C A S E.

January 2d, 1785. Mrs. S——, of W——, near Kidderminfter, aged 38, has been affected with dropfical fwellings of her legs and thighs, about fix weeks, which have gradually grown worfe; has now great difficulty in breathing, which is much increafed on moving; a very irregular, intermittent pulfe, urine in very fmall quantity, and in the feventh month of her pregnancy: a woman of very delicate conftitution, with tender lungs from her infancy, and very fubject to long continued coughs.

R. Pulv. fcillæ gr. iii.
Jalap gr. x. fyr. rofar. folut. tinct. fenn. aa ʒii. aq. menth. v. fimpl. ʒifs. m. mane fumend.

R. pulv. fcillæ Əi. G. ammoniac. fapon. venet. aa sifs. fyr. q. f. f. pilul. 4ª cap. iii. nocte maneque.

On the 7th found her worfe, and the fwelling increafed; the urine about ʒx in the twenty-four hours.

R. Fol. ficcat. Digital. ʒiii. coque in. aq. fontan. ʒxii. ad ʒvi. cola et adde. aq. juniper. comp. ʒii, facchar. alb. ʒfs. m. cap. cochlear. i. larg. 4tis horis.

She

She took about three parts of the medicine before any effect took place. The first was sickness, succeeded by a considerable discharge of urine. She continued the medicine till the whole was consumed, which caused a good deal of sickness for three or four days.

I saw her again on the 12th. The quantity of urine was much increased, and the swelling diminished. Pulse and breathing better.

R. Fol. sicc. Digital. G. assafetid. aa ʒi. calomel. pp. gr. x. sp. lavand. comp. q. s. fiat pilul. xxxii. cap. ii. omni nocte horâ somni.

A plentiful discharge of urine attended the use of these pills, and she got perfectly free from her dropsical complaints.

March 15th she was delivered: had a good labour, was treated as is usual, except in not having her breasts drawn, not intending she should suckle her child, being in so reduced a state. Continued going on well till the 18th, when she was seized with very violent pains across her loins, at times so violent as to make her cry out as much as labour pains. Enema cathartic. Fot. papav. applied to the part.

R. Pulv. ipecacoan. gr. vi. opii. gr. iv. syr. q. s. fiat pilul. vi. capt. i. 2da quaque horâ durante dolore.

H 3   R. Julep.

R. Julep. e camphor. fp. minder. aa ℥ii. capt.
cochlear. i. larg. poſt ſingul. pilul.

19th. Breathing ſhort, unable to lie down, very
irregular low pulſe ſcarcely to be felt, fainty, and
a univerſal cold ſweat: no appetite nor thirſt, ſpaf-
modic pains at times acroſs the loins very violent,
but not ſo frequent as on the preceding day.

R. Gum ammoniac. aſſafetid. aa ʒi. camphor.
gr. xii. fiat pilul. 24. capt. ii. 3tia quaque
hora in cochlear. ii. mixtur. ſeq.

R. Ballam. peruv. 3iii. mucilag. G. arab. q. ſ.
flor. zinci g. vi. aq. menth. ſimp. ℔ſs. m.

Applic. Emp. veſicat. femorib. internis.

R. Sp. vol. fœtid. elixir. paregor. balſam.
Traumatic. aa 3iii. capt. cochlear. parv. ur-
gente languore.

20th. Much the ſame; makes very little water,
and the legs begin to ſwell.—Applic. Emp. e pice
burgund. lumbis.

23d. The ſwelling very much increaſed.—Capt.
gutt. xv. acet. ſcillitic. ter die in two ſpoonfuls of
the following mixture.

R. Infuf. baccar. juniper. ℥vi. tinct. amar. tinct.
ſtomachic. aa ʒi. m.

25th.

25th. Much the fame.

28th. The fwelling confiderably increafed, in other refpects very much the fame.

30th. Breathing very bad, with cough and pain acrofs the fternum, unable to lie down, legs, thighs, and body very much fwelled, urine not more than four or five ounces in the twenty-four hours; hot and feverifh, with thirft.

Applic Emp. veficat. ftomacho et iterno.

R. G. affafetid. ℈ii. pulv. jacob. ℈i. rad. fcill. recent. gr. xii. extract. thebaic. gr. iv. f. pilul. xvi. cap. iv. omni nocte.

R. Sal. nitr. fal. diuretic. aa ʒii. pulv. e contrayerv. comp. ʒi. facchar. ℥i. emulf. commun. ℔i. aq. cinnam. fimpl. ℥i. m. capt. cochlear. iv. ter die.

April 2d. Much the fame, no increafe of urine.

3d. Breathing much relieved by the blifter, which runs profufely. Repeated the medicines, and continued them till the

12th. The cough very bad, pulfe irregular, fwelling much increafed, urine in very fmall quantity, not at all increafed; great lownefs and fainting. She defired to have fome of the pills which relieved

her

her ſo much when with child. I was almoſt afraid to give them, but the inefficacy of the other medicines gave me no hopes of a cure from continuing them, which made me venture to comply with her requeſt.

R. Fol. ſiccat. Digital. G. aſſafetid. aa ʒi. ſp. lavand. comp. q. ſ. f. pilul. xxxii. cap. ii. omni mane; et omni nocte cap. pilul. e ſtyrace gr. vi.

17th. Conſiderable increaſe of urine.

21ſt. Swelling a good deal diminiſhed; urine near four pints in twenty-four hours, which is more than double the quantity ſhe drinks.

Applic. Emp. veſicat. ſemoribus internis.

The Digitalis pills and opiate at bed-time continued. Takes a tea cup of cold chamomile tea every morning.

25th. Swelling much diminiſhed, makes plenty of water, appetite much mended, cough and breathing better. She omitted the medicine for three days; the urine began to diminiſh, the ſwelling and ſhortneſs of breathing worſe. On repeating it for two days, the diſcharge was again augmented, and a diminution of the ſwelling ſucceeded. She has continued the pills ever ſince till the 14th of

May;

May; the dropfical fymptoms and cough are entirely gone, the water is in fufficient quantity, her ftrength is recovered, and fhe has a good appetite. All fhe now complains of is a weight acrofs her ftomach, which is worfe at times, and fhe thinks, unlefs it can be removed, fhe fhall have a return of her dropfy.

Extract of a Letter from Doctor FOWLER, Phyfician, at Stafford.

I UNDERSTAND you are going to publifh on the Digitalis, which I am glad to hear, for I have long wifhed to fee your ideas in print about it, and I know of no one (from the great attention you have paid to the fubject) qualified to treat on it but yourfelf. There are gentlemen of the faculty who give verbal directions to poor patients, for the preparing and taking of an infufion or decoction of the green plant. Would one fuppofe that fuch gentlemen had ever attended to the nature and operation of a fedative power on the functions, *particularly* the *vital?* Is not fuch a vague and unfcientific mode of proceeding putting a two edged fword into the the hands of the ignorant, and the moft likely method to damn the reputation of any very active and powerful medicine? And is it not more than probable that the *neglect* of adhereing to a *certain* and *regular* preparation of the nicotiana, and the *want* (of what you *emphatically* call) a *practicable* dofe, have been the chief caufes of the once rifing reputation of

, **that**

that noted plant being damned above a century ago? In short, the Digitalis is beginning to be used in dropsies, (although some patients are said to go off suddenly under its administration) somewhat in the style of broom ashes; and, in my humble opinion, the public, at this very instant, stand in great need of your *precepts*, *guards*, and *cautions* towards the safe and successful use of such a powerful sedative diuretic; and I have no doubt of your minute attention to those particulars, from a regard to the good and welfare of mankind, as well as to your own reputation with respect to that medicine.

I remember an officer in the Staffordshire militia, who died here of a dropsy five years ago. The Digitalis relieved him a number of times in a wonderful manner, so that in all probability he might have obtained a radical cure, if he would have refrained from hard drinking. I understood it was first ordered for him by a medical gentleman, and its sedative effects proved so mild, and diuretic operation so powerful, that he used to prepare it afterwards for himself, and would take it with as little ceremony as he would his tea. It is said, that he was so certain of its successful operation, that he would boast to his bacchanalian companions, when much swelled, you shall see me in two days time quite another man.

CASES

CASES communicated by Mr. J. FREER, jun. Surgeon, in Birmingham.

C A S E I.

Nov. 1780. Mary Terry, aged 60. Had been subject to asthma for several years; after a severe fit of it her legs began to swell, and the quantity of urine to diminish. In six weeks she was much troubled with the swellings in her thighs and abdomen, which decreased very little when she lay down: she made not quite a pint of water in the twenty-four hours. I ordered her to take two spoonfuls of the infusion of Foxglove every three hours. By the time she had taken eight doses her urine had increased to the quantity of two quarts in the day and night, but as she complained of nausea, and had once vomited, I ordered the use of the medicine to be suspended for two days. The nausea being then removed, she again had recourse to it, but at intervals of six hours. The urine continued to discharge freely, and in three weeks she was perfectly cured of her swellings.

C A S E II.

December, 1782. A poor woman, who had been afflicted with an ague during the whole of her pregnancy, and for two months with dropsical swellings of the feet, legs, thighs, abdomen, and labia pudenda; was at the expiration of the seventh month

taken

taken in labour. On the day after her delivery the ague returned, with so much violence as to endanger her life. As soon as the fit left her, I began to give her the red bark in substance, which had the desired effect of preventing another paroxysm. She continued to recover her health for a fortnight, but did not find any diminution in the swellings; her legs were now so large as to oblige her to keep constantly on the bed, and she made very little water. I ordered her the infusion of Foxglove three times a day, which, on the third day, produced a very copious discharge of urine, without any sickness; she continued the use of it for ten days, and was then able to walk. Having lost all her swellings, and no complaint remaining but weakness, the bark and steel compleated the cure.

Extract of a Letter from Doctor JONES, Physician, in Lichfield.

ANXIOUS to procure authentic accounts from the patients, to whom I gave the Foxglove, I have unavoidably been delayed in answering your last favour. However, I hope the delay will be made up by the efficacy of the plant being confirmed by the enquiry. Long cases are tedious, and seldom read, and as seldom is it necessary to describe every symptom; for every case would be a history of dropsy. I shall therefore content myself with specifying

fying the nature of the difeafe, and when the dropfy is attended with any other affection fhall notice
it.

Two years have fcarcely elapfed fince I firft employed the Digitalis; and the fuccefs I have had
has induced me to ufe it largely and frequently.

C A S E   I.

Ann Willott, 50 years of age, became a patient
of the Difpenfary on the 11th of April 1783. She
then complained of an enlargement of the abdomen, difficulty of breathing, particularly when lying, and coftivenefs. She paffed fmall quantities
of high-coloured urine; and had an evident fluctuation in the belly. Her legs were œdematous.
Chryftals of tartar, fquills, &c. had no effect. The
13th of *June* fhe took two fpoonfuls of a decoction
of Foxglove, containing three drams of the dry
leaves, in eight ounces, three times a day. Her
urine foon increafed, and in a few days fhe paffed
it freely, which continued, and her breath returned.

C A S E   II.

Mr. ———, 45 years of age, had been long
fubject to dropfical fwellings of the legs, and made
little water. Two fpoonfuls of the fame decoction
twice a day, foon relieved him.

CASE

CASE III.

Mrs. ——,aged 70 years. A lady frequently afflicted with the gout, and an asthmatical cough. After a long continuance of the latter, she had a great diminution of urine, and considerable difficulty of breathing, particularly on motion, or when lying. Her body was much bound. There was, however, no apparent swelling. She took three spoonfuls of an aperient decoction of forty-five grains in six ounces and a half, every other morning. The urine was plentiful those days, and her breathing much relieved. In two or three weeks after the use of it she was perfectly restored. The purgative medicine neither increased the urine, nor relieved the breathing, till the Foxglove was added.

This spring she long laboured with the gout in her stomach, which terminated in a fit in her hand. During the whole of this tedious illness, of nearly three months, she passed little urine, and her breathing was again short.

She took the same preparation of Foxglove without any diuretic effect, and afterwards two and three grains of the powder twice a day with as little. The dulcified spirits of vitriol, however, quickly promoted the urinary secretion.

CASE

C A S E   IV.

Mr. C——, 46 years of age, had dropfical fwellings of the legs, and paffed little urine. He took the decoction with three drams, and was foon relieved.

C A S E   V.

Lady ——, took three grains of the dried leaves twice a day, for fwelled legs, and fcantinefs of urine, without effect.

C A S E   VI.

Mrs. Slater, aged 36 years. For dropfy of the belly and legs, and fcantinefs of urine, of feveral weeks ftanding, took three grains of the powder twice a day, and was quite reftored in ten days. She took many medicines without effect.

C A S E   VII.

Mrs. P——, in her 70th year, took three grains of the powder twice a day, for fcantinefs of urine, and fwelled legs, without effect.

C A S E   VIII.

Ann Winterleg, in her 26th year, had dropfical fwellings of the legs, and paffed little urine: fhe was relieved by two drams, in an eight ounce decoction.

CASE

CASE IX.

William Brown, aged 76. In the laſt ſtage of dropſy of the belly and legs, found a conſiderable increaſe of his urine by a decoction of Foxglove, but it was not permanent.

CASE X.

Mr.————, — years of age, and of very groſs habit of body, became highly dropſical, and took various medicines, without effect. One ounce of the decoction, with three drams of the dry leaves in eight ounces, twice or three times a day, increaſed his urine prodigiouſly. He was evidently better, but a little attendant nauſea overcame his reſolution, and in the courſe of ſome weeks afterwards he fell a victim to his obſtinacy.

CASE XI.

Mrs. Smith, about 50 years of age, after a tedious illneſs of many weeks, had a jaundice, and became dropſical in the legs. Two ſpoonfuls of the decoction, with three drams twice a day, increaſed her urine, and abated the ſwelling.

CASE XII.

Widow Chatterton, about 60 years of age. Took the decoction in the ſame way for dropſy of the legs, with little effect.

CASE

CASE XIII.

———— Genders, about thirty-four years of age, was delivered of three children, and became dropfical of the abdomen. She paſſed little or no urine, had conſtant thirſt, and no appetite. She took two ſpoonfuls of an eight ounce decoction, with three drams twice a day. By the time ſhe had finiſhed the bottle, (which muſt have been on the fourth day,) ſhe had evacuated all her water, and could go about. Her appetite increaſed with every doſe, and ſhe recovered without farther help.

CASE . XIV.

Miſs M—— M——, in her 20th year. Had been infirm from her cradle, and, after various ſufferings, had an aſtoniſhing œdematous ſwelling of one leg and thigh, of many weeks ſtanding. She paſſed little or no urine, and had all her other complaints. She took 2 ſpoonfuls of an eight oz. decoction of two drams, twice a day. Her urine immediately increaſed; and, on the third day, the ſwelling had entirely ſubſided.

CASE XV.

Mr. P——, 65 years of age, and of a full habit of body. Had lived freely in his youth, and for many years led rather an inactive life. His health was much impaired ſeveral months, and he had a conſiderable diſtention, and evident fluctuation in

I

the

the abdomen, and a very great œdema of the legs and thighs. His breathing was very short, and rather laborious, appetite bad, and thirst considerable. His belly was bound, and he passed very small quantities of high-coloured urine, that deposited a reddish matter. He had taken medicines some time, and, I believe, the Digitalis; and had been better.

A blister was applied to the upper and inside of each thigh; he took two spoonfuls of the decoction, with three drams of the dry leaves, two or three times a day; and some opening physic occasionally.

He lived at a considerable distance, and I did not visit him a second time; but I was well informed, about ten days or a fortnight afterwards, that his urine increased amazingly upon taking the decoction, and that the water was entirely evacuated.

C A S E   XVI.

Mrs. G——, aged 50 years. After being long ailing, had a large collection of water in the abdomen and lower extremities. Her urine was high-coloured, in small quantities, and had a reddish sediment. She took the decoction of Digitalis, squills, &c. without any effect. The chrystals of tartar, however, cured her speedily.

CASE

CASE XVII.

Mr. ———, about 50 years of age, complained of great tenfion and pain acrofs the abdomen, and of lofs of appetite; his urine, he thought, was lefs than ufual, but the difference was fo trifling he could fpeak with no certainty: his belly feemed to fluctuate. Among other things he tried the Foxglove leaves dried, twice a day; and, although it appeared to afford him relief, yet the effect was not permanent.

CASE XVIII.

Mr. W———, aged between 60 and 70 years; and rather corpulent: was confiderably dropfical, both of the belly and legs, and his urine in finall quantities. Three grains of the dry leaves, twice a day, evacuated the water in lefs than a fortnight.

CASE XIX.

Sarah Taylor, 40 years of age, was admitted into the Difpenfary for dropfy of the abdomen and legs; and was relieved by the Decoctum digitalianum.

CASE XX.

Lydia Smith, aged 60. Difpenfary. Laboured many years under an afthma, and became dropfical. She took the decoction without effect.

CASE

CASE XXI.

John Leadbeater, aged 15 years. Had a quotidian intermittent, which was removed by the humane affiftance of an amiable young lady. His intermittent was foon attended by a very confiderable afcites; for which he became a patient of the Difpenfary. He took a decoction of Foxglove night and morning. His urine increafed immediately, and he loft all his complaints in four days.

CASE XXII.

William Millar, aged 50 years. Admitted into the Difpenfary for a tertian ague, and general dropfy. The dropfy continuing after the ague was removed, and his urine being ftill paffed in fmall quantities; he took the powdered leaves, and recovered his health in five days.

CASE XXIII.

Ann Wakelin, 10 years of age. Had for feveral weeks a dropfy of the belly after an ague. She took a decoction of Foxglove, which removed all complaint by the fourth day.

CASE XXIV.

Ann Meachime; a Difpenfary patient. Had an afcites and fcantinefs of urine. She took the pow-

der

der of Foxglove, and evacuated all her water in three days.

It may not be improper to obferve, 1ft. That various diuretics had long been given in many of thefe cafes before I was confulted. And, 2dly. That the exhibition of the Foxglove was but feldom attended with ficknefs.

REMARKS.

Thefe Cafes, thus liberally communicated by my friend, Dr. Jones, are more acceptable, as they feem to contain a faithful abftract from his notes, both of the unfuccefsful as well as the fuccefsful Cafes.

The following Tabular View of them will give us fome Idea of the efficacy of the Medicine.

Anafarca - - - -	7 Cafes -	Cured - -	3
		Relieved -	1
		Failed - -	3
Afcites - - - -	5 Cafes -	Cured - -	4
		Relieved -	1
Œdematous leg - -	1 Cafe -	Cured - -	1
Afcites and anafarca -	7 Cafes -	Cured - -	4
		Relieved -	2
		Failed - -	1
Afthma and dropfy -	1 Cafe -	Failed - -	1
Hydrothorax and gout	1 Cafe -	Cured - -	1
- - - - -, afcites and anafarca - -	2 Cafes -	Cured - -	2

A CASE

A CASE of Anaſarca communicated by Mr. JONES, Surgeon, in Birmingham.

Dear SIR,

HAVING lately experienced the diuretic powers of the Foxglove, in a caſe of anaſarca; I do myſelf the pleaſure of communicating a ſhort hiſtory of the treatment to you.

I am, &c.

Birmingham,   W. JONES.
May 17th, 1785.

My patient, Mrs. C———, who is in her 51ſt year, had the following ſymptoms, viz. alternate ſwelling of the legs and abdomen, a little cough, ſhortneſs of breath in a morning, thirſt, weak pulſe, and her urine, which was ſo ſmall in quantity as ſeldom to amount to half a pint in twenty-four hours, depoſited a clay-coloured ſediment.

April 16th, 1785, I directed the following form:

R. Fol. Digitalis ſiecat. ʒii.
    Aq. fontanæ bullient. ʒviii. f. infuſ. et cola.
    Sumat cochl. larga iii. o. n. et mane.

On the 17th ſhe had taken twice of the infuſion, and though by miſtake only two tea ſpoonfuls for a doſe, dofe, yet the quantity of urine was increafed to about a pint in the twenty-four hours. She was then directed to take two table fpoonfuls night and morning. And,

On the 18th, a degree of naufea was produced. A pint and half of urine was made in the laft twenty-four hours. During the time above fpecified fhe had two or three ftools every day. The infufion was now omitted.

On the 19th the fwelling of the legs was removed. A degree of naufea took place in the morning, and increafed fo much during the day, that fhe vomitted up all her food and medicine. As fhe was very low, and complained of want of appetite, a cordial julep was directed to be taken occafionally, as well as red port and water, mint tea, &c. She informed me that whatever fhe took generally ftaid about an hour before it came up again, and that the mint tea ftaid longeft on the ftomach. The vomiting decreafed gradually, and ceafed on the 22d. The difcharge of urine remained confiderable during the three following days, but its quantity was not meafured.

22d. A dofe of neutral faline julep was directed to be taken every fourth hour.

On the 23d fhe complained of thirft, and thought the difcharge of urine not fo copious as on the preceding days, therefore the faline julep was continued ed every fourth hour, with the addition of thirty drops of the following medicine:

R. Aceti scillitic. ʒvi.
Tinct. aromat. ʒii.
Tinct. thebaic. gutt. xx. m.

The bowels have been kept open from the 19th, by the occasional use of emollient injections.

On the 24th the legs were much swelled again; she complained of languor and a degree of nausea. The discharge of urine increased a little since the 23d. Her pulse was low and her tongue white. The urine, which had been rendered clear by the infusion of Foxglove, now deposited a whitish sediment.

On the 25th her appetite began to return, the swelling of the legs diminished, and she thought herself much relieved. The urine was considerable in quantity, and clear.

On the 26th she was thirsty and languid. The swelling was removed; the quantity of urine discharged in the last twenty-four hours was about a pint. She continued to mend from this time, and is now in good health.

A giddiness of the head, more or less remarkable at times, was observed to follow the use of the Fox glove, and it lasted nine or ten days.

This

This is the second time that I have relieved this patient by the infusion of Foxglove. I used the same proportion of the fresh leaves the first time as I did of the dried ones the last. The violent vomiting which followed the use of the infusion made with the dried leaves, did not take place with the fresh, though she took near a pint made with the same proportion of the herb fresh gathered.

REMARKS.

THE above is a very instructive case, as it teaches us how small a quantity of the infusion was necessary to effect every desirable purpose. At first sight it may appear from the concluding paragraph, that the green leaves ought to be preferred to the dried ones, as being so much milder in their operation; but let it be noticed, that the same quantity of infusion was prepared from the same weight of the green as of the dried leaves, and consequently, as will appear hereafter, the infusion with the dried leaves was five times the strength of that before prepared from the green ones. We need not wonder, therefore, that the effects of the former were so disagreeable, when the dose was five times greater than it ought to have been. But what makes this matter still more obvious, is the mistake mentioned at first, of two tea spoonfuls only being given for a dose. Now a tea spoonful, containing about a fourth or a fifth part of the contents of a table spoon, the dose then given, was very nearly the same as that which had before been taken of the

infusion

infusion of the green leaves, and it produced precisely the same effects for it increased the urinary discharge, without exciting the violent vomiting.

Letter from Doctor JOHNSTONE, Physician, in Birmingham.

Dear SIR,

THE following cases are selected from many others in which I have given the Digitalis purpurea; and from repeated experience of its efficacy after other diuretics have failed, I can recommend it as an effectual, and when properly managed, a safe medicine.

I am, &c.

Birmingham, May 26,   E. JOHNSTONE.
1785.

March 8th, 1783, I was called to attend Mr. G——, a gentleman of a robust habit, who had led a regular and temperate life, Æt. 68. He was affected with great difficulty of respiration, and cough particularly troublesome on attempting to lie down, œdematous swellings of the legs and thighs, abdomen tense and sore on being pressed, pain striking from the pit of the stomach to the back and shoulders; almost constant nausea, especially after taking food, which he frequently threw up; water thick and high-coloured, passed with difficulty and in

small

small quantity; body costive; pulse natural; face much emaciated, eyes yellow and depressed. He had been subject to cough and difficulty of breathing in the winter for several years; and about four years before this time, after being exposed to cold, was suddenly deprived of his speech and the use of the right side, which he recovered as the warm weather came on; but since that time had been remarkably costive, and was in every.respect much debilitated. He first perceived his legs swell about a year ago; by the use of medicines and exercise, the swellings subsided during the summer, but returned on the approach of winter, and gradually increased to the state in which I found them, notwithstanding he had used different preparations of squills and a great variety of other diuretic medicines. I ordered the following mixture.

R. Foliorum Digitalis purpur. recent. ʒiii. decoque ex aq. fontan. ℥xii ad ℥vi colaturæ adde Tinctur. aromatic.
Syr. zinzib. aa ℥i. m. capt. cochl. duo larga secunda quaque hora ad quartam vicem nisi prius nauseâ supervenerit.

March 9th. He took four doses of the mixture without being in the least sick, and made, during the night upwards of two quarts of natural coloured water.

10th.

10th. Took the remainder of the mixture yesterday afternoon and evening, and was sick for a short time, but made nearly the same quantity of water as before, the swellings are considerably diminished, his appetite increased, but he is still costive.

R. Argent. viv. bolsam peruv. aa ʒss tere ad extinctionem merc. et adde gum. ammon. Ꙅiii aloes socotorin. ʒss rad. scil. recent. Ɇss syr. simpl. q. s. f. mass. in pil. xxxii divid. cap. iii. bis in die.

14th. Continues to make water freely. The swellings of his legs have gradually decreased, soreness and tension of the abdomen considerably less.

Omittant. pil. cap. mistur. c. decoct. Digitalis. &c. ʒtia quaque hora ad ʒtiam vicem.

15th. Made a pint and a half of water last night, without being in the least sick, and is in every respect considerably better. Repet. Pillul. ut antea.

21st. Makes water as usual when in health, and the swellings are entirely gone.

R. Infus. amar. ʒv. tinctur. Rhei spirit. ʒii. spirit vitriol. dulc. ʒii. syr. zinzib. ʒvi. m. cap. cochl. iii. larg. ter in die.

He soon gained sufficient strength to enable him to go a journey, and returned home in much better
health

health than he had been from the time he was affected with the paralytic stroke, and excepting some return of his asthmatic complaint in the winter, hath continued so ever since.

C A S E II.

R——— Howgate, a man much addicted to intemperance, particularly in the use of spirituous liquors, Æt. 60, was admitted into the Hospital near Birmingham, *May* 17, 1783. He complained of difficulty of breathing, attended with cough, particularly troublesome on lying down; drowsiness and frequent dozing, from which he was roused by startings, accompanied with great anxiety and oppression about the breast; oedematous swellings of the legs; constant desire to make water, which he passed with difficulty, and only by drops; pulse weak and irregular; body rather costive; face much emaciated; no appetite for food.—Cap. pil. scil. iii. ter in die.*

May 20th. The pills have had no effect.—Cap. mistur. c. † Decoct. Digital. &c. cochl. ii. larg. 3tia quaque hora, ad 3tiam vicem.

May 21st. Made near two quarts of water in the night, without being in the least sick. He contiued
                                           the

---

* R. Rad. scil. recent. sapon. castiliens. pulv. Rhei opt. aa. ℈i. ol. junip. gutt. xvi. syr. balf. q. s. f. mass. in pil. xxiv. divid.

† Prepared in the same manner as in the former case.

the use of the mixture three times in the day till the 30th, and made about three pints of water daily, by which means the swellings were entirely taken away ; and his other complaints so much relieved, that on the 6th of June he was dismissed free from complaint, except a slight cough. But returning to his old course of life, he hath had frequent attacks of his disorder, which have been always removed by using the Digitalis.

Extract of a letter from Mr. Lyon, Surgeon, at Tamworth.

—Mr. Moggs was about 54 years of age, his disease a dropsy of the abdomen, attended with anasarcous swellings of the limbs, &c. brought on by excessive drinking. I believe the first symptoms of the disease appeared the beginning of November, 1776 ; the medicines he took before you saw him, were squills in different forms, sal diureticus and calomel, but without any good effect ; he begun the Digitalis on the 10th of July 1777 ; a few doses of it caused a giddiness in the head, and almost deprived him of sight, with very great nausea, but very little vomiting, after which a considerable flow of urine ensued, and in a very short time, a very little water remained either in the cavity of the abdomen, or the membrana adiposa, but he remained excessive weak, with a fluttering pulse at the rate of 150 or frequently 160 in a minute ; he kept pretty free from water for upwards of twelve months ; it then

collect-

collected, and neither the Digitalis nor any other medicine would carry it off. I tapped him the 2d of Auguſt 1779 in the uſual place, and took ſome gallons of water from him, but he very ſoon filled again, and as he had a very large rupture, a conſiderable quantity of the water lodged in the ſcrotum, and could not be got away by tapping in the uſual place. I therefore (on the 28th of the ſame month) made an inciſion into the lower part of the ſcrotum, and drained off all the water that way, but he was ſo very much reduced, that he died the 8th or 9th of *September* following, which was about two years and two months after he firſt begun the Digitalis.

I have had ſeveral dropſical patients relieved, and ſome perfectly recovered by the Digitalis, ſince you attended Mr. Meggs, but as I did not take any notes or make any memorandums of them, cannot give you any of them.

Communications from Dr. STOKES, Phyſician, in Stourbridge.

Dear SIR,

I ACCEPT with pleaſure your invitation to communicate what I know reſpecting the properties of *Digitalis*; and if an account of what others had diſcovered before you,* with a deTail

---

* See this account in the Introduction.

tail of my own experience, fhall be allowed the merit of at leaft a well meant acknowledgment, for the early communication you were fo kind to make me, of the valuable properties you had found in it; I fhall confider my time as well employed. A knowledge of what has been already done is the beft ground work of future experiment; on which account I have been the more full on this fubject, in hopes that given with the cautions which you mean to lay down in the cure of dropfies, it may prove alike ufeful in that of other difeafes, one of which ftands foremoft among the *opprobria* of medicine.

C A S E   I.

Mrs. M——. Orthopnea, pain, and exceffive oppreffion at the bottom of the fternum. Pulfe irregular, with frequent intermiffions. Appetite very much impaired. Legs anafarcous.

Empl. veficator. pectori dolent.
Infuf. Digital. e ʒiii. ad. aq. &c. ʒviii. cochl. j. o.
h. donec naufea excitetur vel diurefis fatis copi-
ofa proveniat.

I ordered it of the above ftrength, and to be repeated often, on account of the great emergency of the cafe, but the naufea excited by the firft dofe prevented its being given at fuch fhort intervals. A 3d dofe I found had been given, which was followed by vomitings. All her complaints gradually abated, bu but in about a fortnight recurred, notwithſtanding the uſe of infuſ. amar. &c.

Dec. 2. Infus. Digit. e. ʒiſs ad aq. &c. ℨviii. cochl. ii. horis &c. u. a.

Complaints gradually abated, ſwellings of the legs nearly gone down.

About a month afterwards you was deſired to viſit this patient.＊

———————————

＊ For reaſons aſſigned at p. 100, I did not intend to introduce any caſe, occuring under my own inſpection, in the courſe of the preſent year ; but it may be ſatisfactory to continue the hiſtory of this diſeaſe, as Dr. Stokes's narrative would otherwiſe be incomplete.

1785.

C A S E.

Jan. 5th. Mrs. M——, Æt. 48. Hydrothorax and anaſarcous legs, of eight months duration. She had taken jallap, ſquill, ſalt of tartar, and various other medicines. I found her in a very reduced ſtate, and therefore directed only a grain and half of the Pulv. Digital. to be given night and morning. This in a few days encreaſed the ſecretion of urine, removed her difficulty of breathing, and reduced the ſwelling of her legs, without any diſturbance to her ſyſtem.

Three months afterwards, a ſevere attack of gout in her legs and arms, removing to her head, ſhe died.

Dr. Stokes had an opportunity of examining the dead body, and I had the ſatisfaction to learn from him, that there did not appear to have been any return of the dropſy.

K   On

On the examination of the body I noticed, among others, the following appearances.

About ½ oz. of bloody water flowed out, on elevating the upper half of the ſcull, and a ſmall quantity alſo was found at the baſe.

BRAIN. Blood-veſſels turgid with blood, and many of thoſe of conſiderable ſize diſtended with air.

A very ſlight watery effuſion between the *Pia Mater* and *Tunica arachnoidea.* About ¼ oz. of watery fluid in the *lateral ventricles.*

THORAX. In the left cavity about 4 oz. of bloody ſerum; in the right but little. Lungs, the hinder parts loaded with blood. Adheſions of each lobe to the pleura. *Pericardium* containing but a very ſmall quantity of fluid. *Heart* containing no coagula of blood. *Valves of the Aorta* of a cartilaginous texture, as if beginning to oſſify.

Abdominal Viſcera natural, and a profuſion of *Fat* under the integuments of the abdomen and thorax, in the former to the thickneſs of an inch and upwards, and in very conſiderable quantity on the meſentery, omentum, kidneys, &c.

OBS. The intermitting pulſe ſhould ſeem to have been owing to effuſions of water in ſome of the cavities of the breaſt, as it diſappeared on the removal of the waters.

CASE

C A S E II.

Mrs. C—— of K————, Æt. 80. Orthopnœa, with sense of oppression about the præcordia. Unable to lie down in bed for some nights past. Anasarca of the lower extremities. Urine very scanty. Complaints of six weeks standing. Had taken *sal. diuret. c. ol. junip.—Calom. c. jalap, et gambog.—Et ol. junip. c. ol. Terebinth.* without effect.

Feb. 7. *Infus. Digital. c. ʒiii. ad aq. &c. ℥viii. cochl. ii. 4tis horis.* Ordered to drink largely of *infus. baccar. junip.* The third dose produced great nausea which continued ten hours, during which time the urine made was about a quart. The next day her apothecary directed her to begin again with it. The second dose produced vomiting. During the next twenty hours she made two quarts of water, about four times as much as she drank.

From this time she took no more of the *infus. Digital.* but continued the *inf. bacc. junip.* until about *March* 2d, when all the swellings were gone down, her respiration perfectly free, and she herself quite restored to her former state of health. On the 29th she had an attack of jaundice which was some time after removed; since which she has enjoyed a good state of health, excepting that for some little time past her ancles have been slightly œdematous, which will I trust soon yield to strengthening medicines.

K 2   CASE

C A S E   III.

Mrs. M—— G——, Æt. 64. Has had fore legs for thefe thirty-four years paft. Orthopnœa. Senfe of oppreffion at the præcordia. Pulfe intermitting. Legs anafarcous. Urine fcanty, high-coloured.

> *Infus. Digital. c. ʒifs ad aq. bull. ℥viii. cochl. ii.*
> *4tis horis.*

Took fix dofes, when naufea was excited. Urine a quart during the courfe of the night. The flow of urine continued, and complaints relieved. Sal. Mart. c. extr. gent. and afterwards with the addition of extr. cort. for which laft ingredient fhe had a predilection, confirmed the cure.

On the fame day the next year I was called in to her for a fimilar train of fymptoms, excepting that the pulfe was but juft perceptibly irregular.

> *Infus. Digital. u. a. præfcript.*

The directions on the phial not being attended to, *two dofes of it were given after a naufea had been excited*, which, with occafional vomitings, became exceedingly oppreffive. A faline draught, given in Dr. Hulme's method, a draught *fal. c. c. gr. aii. c. conf. card. gr. x.* produced no immediate effect, but the naufea gradually abating, inf. bacc. junip. was ordered; but this appeared to augment it,
and

and a great propensity to sleep coming on, I directed *sal. c. c. conf. card. aa gr. viii. Alis horis*, which removed the unpleasant symptoms and *myrrh. c. sal. mart.* completed the cure. During the use of the above medicines, the urine was augmented, and the pulmonary complaints removed, even before the nausea left her; and the sores of her legs which were much inflamed before she began with the infuf. Digital. in a day's time assumed a much healthier appearance, and on her other complaints going off, they shewed a greater tendency to heal than she had ever observed in them for twenty years before. This instance is a very pleasing confirmation of the experience of Hulse and Dr. Baylies, and of the advantage to be derived from a medicine, which, while it helps to heal the ulcers, removes that from the constitution which often renders the healing of them improper.

In one case in which I ordered it, the infusion, instead of digesting three hours as I had directed, was suffered to stand upon the leaves all night. The consequence was that the first dose produced considerable nausea.

The two following cases, with which I have been favoured by a physician very justly eminent, convince me of the necessity there is that every one who discovers a new medicine, or new virtues in an old one, should, in announcing such discoveries, publish to the world the exact manner in which he exhi-

bits

bits fuch medicines, with all the precautions neceffary to obtain the promifed fuccefs.

In thefe (fays my correfpondent) " the infufion
" was given in fmall dofes, repeated every hour or
" two, till a naufea was raifed, when it was omit-
" ted for a day or perhaps two, and then repeated
" in the fame manner."

" An Ascites emptied by it, but filled again
" very fpeedily, though *its ufe was never difconti-*
" *nued,* and who afterwards found no falutary ef-
" fects from it.   Ended fatally."

" In an Anasarca it fometimes increafed the
" quantity of urine, and abated the fwelling, but
" which as often returned in as great a degree as
" before, though *the medicine was ftill given,* and al-
" ways increafed in quantity fo as to excite naufea.
" Ended fatally."

" I have tried it in many other cafes, but found
" very little difference in the fuccefs attending it."

May we not be allowed to conjecture that the inefficacy of *its continued ufe* is owing to its narcotic property gradually diminifhing the irritability of the
mufcular fibres of the abforbents, or poffibly of the
whole vafcular fyftem, and thus adding to that
weakened action which feems to be the caufe of the
generality of dropfies, which leads us to caution
the medical experimenter againft trying it, at leaft

againft

againſt its continued uſe, even in ſmall doſes, in other diſeaſes of diminiſhed energy, as continued fever, palſy, &c.

I remain with the greateſt truth,

Your obliged and affectionate friend,

Stourbridge,   JONATHAN STOKES.
May 17, 1785.

THE three following Hoſpital Caſes, which Dr. STOKES had an opportunity of obſerving, are related as inſtances of bad practice, and tend to demonſtrate how neceſſary it is when one phyſician adopts the medicine of another, that he ſhould alſo at firſt rigidly adopt his method.

C A S E   I.

Eſther K——, Æt. 33. General anaſarca, aſcites, and dyſpnœa, of ſeven months duration.

Decoct. e Digit. ʒiv. c. aq. ℔i. coquend. ad ℔ſs. cap. ʒi. 2dis. horis. 1ſt DAY. 4th doſe made her ſick. 2d DAY. The firſt doſe ſhe took to-day produced vomiting.

3d DAY.

3d Day. *Minuatur dofis ad ʒ ſs.* This ſtayed upon her ſtomach, but produced an almoſt conſtant ſickneſs. Stools more frequent, water ſcarce ſenſibly increaſed; and her ſwellings not at all reduced.

4th Day. *Cap. Calomel. gambog. ſcill. &c.*

Obs. Sufficient time was not allowed to obſerve its effects, neither was the patient enjoined the free uſe of diluents. The diſeaſe terminated fatally.

C A S E   II.

William T——, Æt. 42. Aſcites, with cough and dyſpnœa. Abdomen very much diſtended. The reſt of his body highly emaciated. Urine thick, high coloured, and in very ſmall quantity.

Decoct Digit. (u. in Eſther K——,) 4tis horis.

1ſt Day of taking it. The 4th doſe produced ſickneſs.

2d. Vomiting after the ſecond doſe.

10th. Urine increaſed to ℔vi.

11th. Flow of urine continues. Abdomen quite flaccid.

12th. Ab-

12th. Abdomen not diminifhed.

15th. A fmart purging came on, and the flow of urine diminifhed.

23d. Belly much bound. Took a cathart. powder, which was followed by a diminution of the abdomen.

29th. To take a cathart. powder every 4th morning, continuing the decoct. Digit.

32d. Urine exceedingly fcanty.

35th. *Vin. fcill. ʒfs. o. m. &c.* This produced diuretic effects.

44th. Tapped. Terminated fatally.

Obs. Here the medicine was *continued till it ceafed to produce diuretic effects;* and thefe effects were not aided by any ftrengthening remedies.

C A S E   III.

George R——, Æt. 52. Afcites, general anafarca, and dyfpnœa. His legs fo greatly diftended that it was with great difficulty he could draw the one after the other.

Infuf.

Infuf. Digital. ʒiiiſs. ad. aq. foſs. cap. ʒi. altern. horis donec nauſeam excitaverit. Rep. ʒtiis diebus. tempore intermedio cap. ſol. guaic. ʒi. ter in die ex inf. ſinap.

1ſt Day of taking it. Became ſickiſh towards night.

2d Day. Made a great quantity of water during the night, and ſpat up a great deal of watery phlegm. The firſt doſe he took in the morning has produced a ſickneſs which has continued all day, but he has never vomited.

3d. Day. The change in his appearance ſo great as to make it difficult to conceive him to be the ſame perſon. Inſtead of a large corpulent man, he appeared tall, thin, and rather aged. Breathes freely, and can walk up and down ſtairs without inconvenience.

4th Day. *Decoſt. bacc. junip. and cyder for common drink.*

6th Day. A ſecond courſe of his medicine produced a flow of urine almoſt as plentiful as the former, though he drank little or nothing at the time. In a day or two after he walked to ſome diſtance.

12th Day. *Pot. purgans illico.*

14th Day. *Pot. purg. c. jalap. ʒſs. 4tis diebus. Infuf. Dig. ʒtiis diebus.*

17th Day.

17th Day. *R. Gamb. gr. iii. calom. gr. ii. camph. gr. i. fyr. fimpl. fiat pil. o. n. fum. Infuf. Digit. ʒtiis diebus.*

21ft Day.   Made an out-patient.   The super-abundant flow of urine continued for the firft three days after his laft courfe ; but fince, the flow of faliva has been nearly equal to that of urine.

The fmalls of his legs not quite reduced, and are fuller at night.   He has fhrunk round the middle from four feet two inches to three feet fix inches ; and in the calves of his legs, from feventeen inches to thirteen and a half.*

Obs. The waters were here very fuccefsfully evacu-ated, but as you remarked to me, on communicat-ing the cafe to you at the time, tonic medicines fhould have been given, to fecond the ground that had been gained, inftead of weakening the patient by draftic purgatives.

----

* In the three laft recited cafes, the medicine was directed in dofes quite too ftrong, and repeated too frequently. If Efther K—— could have furvived the extreme ficknefs, the diuretic effects would probably have taken place, and, from her time of life, I fhould have expected a recovery. Wm. T —— feems to have been a bad cafe, and I think would not have been cured un-der any management.   G. R—— certainly poffeffed a good con-ftitution, or he muft have fhared the fate of the other two.

A CASE

A CASE from Mr. Shaw, Surgeon, at
Stourbridge. — Communicated by Doctor
Stokes.

Matth. D——, Æt. 71. Tall and thin. Difeafe a
general anafarca, with great difficulty of breathing.
The lac ammoniac. fomewhat relieved his breath ;
but the fwellings increafed, and his urine was not
augmented.   I confidered it as a loft cafe, but having feen the good effects of the Digitalis, as ordered
by Dr. Stokes in the cafe of Mrs. G——, I gave
him one fpoonful of an infufion of ʒii. to half a pint,
twice a day.   His breath became much eafier, his
urine increafed confiderably, and the fwellings gradually difappeared; fince which his health has been
pretty good, except that about three weeks ago, he
had a flight dyfpnœa, with pain in his ftomach,
which were foon removed by a repetition of the
fame medicine.

Mr. Shaw likewife informs me, that he has removed pains in the ftomach and bowels, by giving
a fpoonful of the infufion, ʒifs. to ℥viii. morning
and night.

A Letter

A Letter from Mr. V A U x, Surgeon, in Birmingham.

Dear SIR,

I SEND you the two following cafes, wherein the Digitalis had very powerful and fenfible effects, in the cure of the different patients.

C A S E I.

Mrs. O—— of L—— ftreet, in this town, aged 28, naturally of a thin, fpare habit, and her family inclinable to phthifis, fent for me on the 11th of June, 1779, at which time fhe complained of great pain in her fide, a conftant cough, expectorated much, which funk in water; had colliquative fweats and frequent purging ftools; the lower extremities and belly full of water, and from the great difficulty fhe had in breathing, I concluded there was water in the cheft alfo. The quantity of water made at a time for three weeks before I faw her, never amounted to more than a tea-cup full, frequently not fo much. Finding her in fo alarming a fituation, I gave it as my opinion fhe could receive no benefit from medicine, and requefted her not to take any; but fhe being very defirous of my ordering her fomething, I complied, and fent her a box of gum pills with fquills, and a mixture with falt of tartar: thefe medicines fhe took until the fixteenth, without any good effects: the water in her legs now began to ex-
fude

sude through the skin, and a small blister on one of her legs broke. Believing she could not exist much longer, unless an evacuation of the water could be procured; after fully informing her of her situation, and the uncertainty of her surviving the use of the medicine, I ventured to propose her taking the Digitalis, which she chearfully agreed to. I accordingly sent her a pint mixture, made as under, of the fresh leaves of the Digitalis. Three drams infused in one pint of boiling water, when cold strained off, without pressing the leaves, and two ounces of the strong juniper water added to it: of this mixture she was ordered four table spoonfulls every third hour, till it either made her sick, purged her, or had a sensible effect on the kidneys. This mixture was sent on the seventeenth, and she began taking it at noon on the eighteenth. At one o'clock the following morning I was called up, and informed she was dying. I immediately attended her, and was agreeably surprised to find their fright arose from her having fainted, in consequence of the sudden loss of twelve quarts of water she had made in about two hours. I immediately applied a roller round her belly, and, as soon as they could be made, 2 others, which were carried from the toes quite up the thighs. The relief afforded by these was immediate; but the medicine now began to affect her stomach so much, that she kept nothing on it many minutes together. I ordered her to drink freely of beef tea, which she did, but kept it on her stomach but a very short time. A neutral draught in a state of effervescence was taken to no good purpose: She therefore continued
the

the beef tea, and took no other medicine for five days, when her sickness went off : her cough abated, but the pain in her side still continuing, I applied a blister which had the desired effect : her urine after the first day flowed naturally. Her cure was compleated by the gum pills with steel and the bitter infusion. It must be observed she never had any collection of water afterwards.

It affords me great pleasure to inform you that she is now living, and has since had four children ; all of whom, I think I may justly say, are indebted to the Digitalis for their existence.

There appears in this case a striking proof of the utility of emetics in some kinds of consumptions, as it appears to me the dropsy was brought on by the cough, &c. and I believe these were cured by the continual vomitings, occasioned by the medicine.

C A S E   II.

Mr. H——, a publican, aged about 48 years, sent for me in *March*, 1778. He complained of a cough, shortness of breathing, which prevented him from laying down in bed ; his belly, thighs and legs very much distended with water ; the quantity of urine made at a time seldom exceeded a spoonful. I requested him to get some of the Digitalis, and as they had no proper weights in the house, I told them to put as much of the fresh leaves as would weigh down a guinea, into half a pint of boiling water :

to

to let it stand till cold, then to pour off the clear liquor, and add a glass of gin to it, and to take three table spoonfuls every third hour, until it had some sensible effect upon him.

Before he had taken all the infusion, the quantity of urine made increased, (he therefore left off taking it), and it continued to do so until all the water was evacuated. His breathing became much better, his cough abated, though it never quite left him : he being for some time before asthmatic. By taking some tonic pills he continued quite well until the next spring, when he had a return of his complaint, which was carried off by the same means. Two years after, he had a third attack, and this also gave way to the medicine. Last year he died of a pleurisy.

I am, &c.

Moor-Street, 8th May,　　　JER. VAUX.
1785.

P, S. You must well recollect the case of Mrs. F——.—It was " a general dropsy—every time " she took the medicine its effects were similar, viz. " The discharge of urine came on gradually at first, " increased afterwards, and the whole of the water " both in the belly, legs, &c. was perfectly evacuated. " Although the effects were only temporary, they " were exceedingly agreeable to the patient, making " her time much more comfortable."—— (See Case XLIII.)

A Let-

A Letter from Mr. WAINWRIGHT, Surgeon,
in Dudley.

Dear Sir,

IT gives me great pleasure to
find you intend to publish your observations on
the Digitalis purpurea.

Several years are now elapsed since you communicated to me the high opinion you entertained of
the diuretic qualities of this noble plant. To ensure
success, due attention was recommended to its *preparation*, its *dose*, and its *effects* upon the system.

I always gave the infusion of the dried leaves;
the dose the same as in the prescriptions returned.
If the medicine operated on the stomach or bowels,
it was thought prudent to forbear. When the kidneys began to perform their proper functions, and
the urine to be discharged, a continuance of its farther use was unnecessary.

These remarks you made in the case of the first
patient for whom you prescribed the Digitalis in our
neighbourhood, and I have found them all necef-
sary at this present period. From the *decided* good effects
that followed from its use, in those cases where the
most powerful remedies had failed, I was soon convinced it was a most valuable addition to the materia
medica.

L　　　　　　　Th

The want of a certain diuretic, has long been one of the defiderata of medicine. The Digitalis is undoubtedly at the head of that clafs, and will feldom, if properly adminiftered, difappoint the expectation. I can fpeak with the more confidence, having, in an extenfive practice, been a happy witnefs to its good qualities.

For feveral years, I have given the infufion in a variety of cafes, where there was a deficiency in the fecretion of the urine, with the greateft fuccefs. In recent obftructions, I do not recollect many failures. In anafarcous difeafes, and in the anafarca, when combined with the afcites ; in fwellings of the limbs, and in difeafes of the cheft, when there was the greateft reafon to believe an accumulation of ferum, the moft beneficial confequences have followed from its ufe.

Had I been earlier acquainted with your intention to publifh an account of the Digitalis, I could have tranfmitted fome cafes, which might have ferved to corroborate thefe affertions : but I am convinced the Digitalis needs not my affiftance to procure a favorable reception. Its own merit will enfure fuccefs, more than a hundred recited cafes.

I could wifh thofe gentlemen who intend to make ufe of this plant, to collect it in a hot dry day, when the petals fall, and the feed-veffels begin to fwell.

The

The leaves kept to the second year are weaker, and their diuretic qualities much diminished. It will therefore be necessary to gather the plant fresh every season.

These cautions are unnecessary to the accurate botanist, who well knows, that a plant in the spring, though more succulent and full of juices, is destitute of those qualities which may be expected when that plant has attained its full vigour, and the seed-vessels begin to be manifest. But for want of attention to these particulars, its virtues may be thought exaggerated, or doubtful, if beneficial consequences do not always flow from its use. There are diseases it cannot cure; and in several of those patients in this town, who first took the Digitalis by your orders, there was the most positive proof of the viscera being unsound. In these desperate cases it often procured a plentiful flow of urine, and palliated a disease which mecine could not remove.

At a remote distance, physicians are seldom applied to for advice in trifling disorders. Many remedies have been tried without relief, and the disease is generally obstinate or confirmed. — It would not be fair to try the merits of the Digitalis in this scale. It might often fail of promoting the end desired. I flatter myself the reputation of this plant will be equal to its merit, and that it will meet with a candid reception.

As

As there is no pleasure equal to relieving the miseries and distresses of our fellow-creatures, I hope you will long enjoy that peculiar felicity.

Permit me to return my thankful acknowledgments, for your free communication of a medicine, by which means, through the blessing of providence, I have been enabled to restore health and happiness to many miserable objects.

I am, &c.

Yours,

Dudley, April 26th,   J. WAINWRIGHT
1785.

CASE of Mr. WARD, Surgeon, in Birmingham.—Related by himself.

IN *September*, 1782, I was seized with a difficulty of breathing, and oppression in my chest, in consequence of taking cold from being called out in the night. My tongue was foul; my urine small in quantity; my breath laborious and distressing on the slightest exercise. I tried the medicines most generally recommended, such as emetics, blisters, lac ammoniacum, oxymel of squills. &c but finding little or no relief, I consulted Dr. Withering, who advised me to try the following prescription.

R. Fol

R. Fol. Digital. purp. ficcat. ʒifs.
Aq. bullientis ʒiv.
Aq. cinn. fp. ʒfs. digere per horas quatuor,
et colaturæ capiat cochlear. i. nocte maneque.

He alfe defired me to take fifty drops of tincture
of cantharides three or four times a day.

After taking eight ounces of the infulion, and
about twelve drams of the drops, I was perfectly
cured, and have had no return fince. The medicine did not occafion ficknefs or vertigo, nor had
they any other fenfible effect than in changing the
appearance, and increafing the quantity of the urine,
and rendering the tongue clean. After the laſt dofe
or two indeed, I had a little naufea, which was immediately removed by a fmall glafs of brandy.

Birmingham, 1ſt July, 1785.

Communications from Mr. YONGE, Surgeon, in Shiffnall, Shropſhire.

Dear Sɪʀ,

I HAVE great fatisfaction in
complying with your juſt claim, by tranfcribing out-
lines of the fubfequent cafes for infertion in your long
requeſted tract on the Digitalis purpurea. The two
firſt of thefe you will eafily recollect, the cures having
been conducted immediately under your own manage-
L 3 ment

ment, and the whole may add to that weight of evidence which long experience enables you to adduce of the efficacy of that valuable medicine. I have recited the only instances of its failure which occur to me, but many other, though successful cases, wherein its utility might seem dubious, and also the accounts received from people whose accuracy might be suspected, I shall not for obvious reasons trouble you with.

I am, dear Sir,

Your obliged friend,

Shiffnall,　　　　　　WILLIAM YONGE.
May 1, 1785.

C A S E I.

A Gentleman aged 49, on the night of the 21st of August, 1784, awaked with a sense of suffocation, which obliged him to rise up suddenly in bed. I found him complaining of difficult respiration, particularly on lying down; the countenance pale, and the pulse smaller and quicker than usual. Some brandy and water having been given, the symptoms gradually abated, so that he slept in a half recumbent posture. The following day he expressed a sense of anxiety and weight in the chest, attended by quicker breathing upon motion of the body. That evening an emetic of ipecacohana was given, and afterwards a draught, with vitriolic æther
and

and confect. card. aa ʒ to be repeated as the symptoms should require it. He continued to be affected with slighter returns of the dyspnœa at irregular intervals, until *September* 15th, when upon a more severe attack, the emetic was repeated. He now recollected some slight pain in his arms which had affected him previous to this last seizure, and was disposed to consider his complaint as rheumatic. Pills with gum ammoniac. gum guaiac. and antimonial powder were directed, with infus. amar. simpl. twice a day. The bowels were regulated by aperient pills of pulv. jalap. aloes and sal. tartar. and ʒiss balsam peruv. was given occasionally to alleviate the paroxysms of dyspnœa.

From this period until the beginning of November, little amendment or variation happened, except that respiration became more permanently difficult, and particularly oppressed upon motion, nor was it relieved by the expectoration of a mucous discharge, which now increased considerably. Squills, musk, ol. succini, æther, with other medicines of the same kind, were now used, but without success. The effects of opium and venæsection were tried. The appetite diminished, and his sleep became short and disturbed. He sometimes slept lying upon his back, but generally upon his left side. The urine which had hitherto been of good colour, and sufficient quantity, now became diminished, and lateritious; and the ancles œdematous.

On

On the 15th of *November* a blister was laid over the sternum, and ʒiss of oxymel scillitic. was given every eight hours.

On the 18th, a more copious discharge of urine took place; the swelling of the feet soon disappeared, and the respiration became gradually relieved.

On the 30th ʒi tinct. cantharidum twice a day in pyrmont water, with pills of ammoniac, sal tartar. et extract. gentian. were substituted, but

On the 7th of *December*, from some symptoms of relapse, the oxymel was used as before, and continued to be taken until the 27th, in doses as large as could be dispensed with on account of the great nausea which attended its exhibition: The urine was made in the quantity of four or five pints each day, during the whole time; the quantity then drank being seldom more than three pints. But now the sickness being exceedingly depressing, the strength failing, and the diuretic effects beginning to cease, the following prescription was directed.

R. Fol. Digitalis purpur. pulv. ʒss.
Spec. Aromatic. ʒi. sp. lav. c. f. pilul. no. x. capiat i. nocte maneque, et alternis diebus sensim augeatur dosin.

In three days the effect of this medicine became sible, and when the dose of the Digitalis had been
increased

increased to six grains per day, the flow of urine generally amounted to seven pints every twenty-four hours. Not the least sickness, nor any other disagreeable symptom supervened, though he persevered in this plan until the end of *January* at which time the dyspnœa was removed, and he has continued gradually to regain his flesh, strength, and appetite, without any relapse.

C A S E   II.

About the middle of the year 1784 a lady aged 48, returned from London, to her native air in Shropshire, under symptoms of complicated disease. It was your opinion that the plethoric state, consequent to that period, when menstruation first begins to cease, had under various appearances, laid the foundation of that deplorable state which now presented itself. The skin was universally of a pale, leaden colour; her person much emaciated, and her strength so reduced, as to disable her from walking without support. The appetite fluctuating, the digestion impaired so much, that solids passed the intestines with little appearance of solution : She had generally eight or ten alvine evacuations every day, and without this number, febrile symptoms, attended with severe vertiginous affection, and vomiting regularly ensued. The stools were of a pale ash colour. The urine generally pale, and at first in due quantity. The region of the stomach had

had a tenfe feel, without forenefs: the feet and
ancles œdematous, her fleep was uncertain: the
pulfe varying between 94 and 100, and feeble,
except upon the approach of the menftrual periods,
which were now only marked by its increafed
ftrength, and exacerbation of other febrile fymptoms. Emetics, faline medicines, and gentle aperients were neceffary to alleviate thefe. Six grains
of ipecac. operated with fufficient power, and half
a grain of calomel would have purged with great
violence.

From the time of her arrival till the middle of
Auguft, mercury had been continued in various
forms, and in dofes fuch as the irritable ftate of her
ftomach and bowels would admit of. Spirit. nitri
dulc.; fal. tartar. fquill, and cantharides were
alternately employed as diuretics, but without fuccefs, to retard the progrefs of an univerfal anafarca,
which was then advanced to fuch degree and accompanied by fo great debility, and other dreadful con-
comitants, as to threaten a fpeedy and fatal cataf-
trophe.

On the 16th of *Auguft* you firft faw her, and
directed thus.

R. Mercur. cinerei gr. ii.
Fol. Digital. purpur. pulv. ɘi. f. mafs. in
pill. no. xvi. dividend.—fumat unam hora meridia-
ana, iterumque hora quinta pomeridiana quotidie.

Capiat

Capiat lixivii faponac. gutt. L. in hauft. jufcul. fine fale parati omni nocte.

On the 20th the flow of urine began to increafe, and fhe continued the medicine in the fame dofe until the 20th of *September*, difcharging from fix to eight pints of water each day for the firft week, and which quantity gradually diminifhed as fhe became empty. During this period fhe complained not of any ficknefs, except from the lixivium, which was after the firft dofe reduced to 20 drops; and her appetite and ftrength increafed daily, though it was evident that no bile had yet flowed into the bowels, nor was the digeftion at all improved. The anafarcous appearances being then removed, the Digitalis was omitted, and pills, compofed of mercur. cinereus, aloes, and fal tartari directed twice a day, with ʒi. of vin. chalybeat. in infuf. amar. fimpl.

Her amendment in other refpects proceeded flowly, but regularly, from that time until the 9th of October; when the ftate of plethora again recurring, with its ufual attendant fymptoms, ʒiv. of blood were taken from the arm; and this was upon the fame occafion, repeated in the following month, with manifeft good confequences; though in both inftances the colour of the blood, as flowing from the vein could hardly be called red, and the coagulum was as weak in its cohefion as poffible. The ftate of the ftomach and bowels was by this time greatly improved, in common with other parts of the

the fyftem; but no intromiffion of bile had yet happened: the hardnefs about the hypogaftric region, though lefs, continued in a confiderable degree, and you ordered pills of mercury rubbed down, and ruft of iron, to be taken twice a day, with a decoction of dandelion and fal fodæ.

A cataplafm of linfeed was applied every night over the ftomach and right fide; and, with little deviation from this plan, fhe continued to the end of the year, improving in her general health, but the hepatic affection yet remaining. It was then determined to try the effects of electricity, and gentle fhocks were paffed through the body daily, and as nearly as could be through the liver, in various directions.

On the fifth day there was reafon to think that fome gall had been fecreted and poured out, and this became every day more evident; but it flowed only in fmall quantity, and irregularly into the bowels, as appeared from the fæces being partially tinged by it.

In *February* the lady left this neighbourhood, and though convalefcent, yet fo nearly well as to promife us the fatisfaction of feeing her perfectly reftored.

June 29. The bile is now fecreted in pretty good quantity, her appetite is perfectly good, her ftrength equal to almoft any degree of exercife, and her

health

health in general better than it has been for some years.

C A S E   III.

Mr. W——, aged —. In *June*, 1782, was affected with flight difficulty in respiration, upon taking exercise or lying down in bed. These symptoms increased gradually until the end of *July*, when he complained of sense of weight and uneasiness about the proecordia; loss of appetite; and costiveness. The urine was small in quantity, and high coloured; his pulse feeble, and intermitting; he breathed with difficulty when in bed, and slept little. After the exhibition of an emetic, and an opening medicine of rhubarb, sena, and sal tartari, he was directed to take half a dram of squill pill, pharm. Edinburg. night and morning, with 3ſs sal. sodæ in ʒiſs. inſuf. amar. ſimpl. twice a day; and these medicines were continued during ten days, without any sensible effect. A blister was then applied to the sternum, and six grains of calomel given in the evening. The symptoms were now increased very considerably, in every particular; and the following infusion was substituted for the former medicines.

R. Fol. Digital. purpur. ʒiii.
    Cort. limon. ʒii. infund.
    Aq. bullient. ℔i. per hor. ♀ et cola. sumat
cochl. i. primo mane et repet. omni hora.

Sometime

Sometime in the night confiderable naufea occurred, and the following day he began to make water in great quantity, which he continued to do for three or four days. The pulfe in a few hours became regular, flower, and ftronger, and, in the courfe of a week, all the fymptoms entirely vaniſhed, and an electuary of cort. peruvian, fal martis, and fpec. aromatic. confirmed his cure.

In *February*, 1784, this gentleman had a relapfe of his difeafe, from which he again foon recovered by the fame means, and is now perfectly well.

CASE IV.

G—— A——, a hufbandman, aged 57. Was in the year 1782 affected with a flight, but conftant pain in his breaft, with difficult refpiration. His countenance was yellow; the abdomen fwelled, and hard; his urine high coloured, and in fmall quantity; appetite and fleep little. Complained of frequent naufea, and of fudden profufe fweatings, which feemed for a ſhort time to relieve the dyfpnœa.

After the exhibition of an emetic, fix grains of calomel were given, with a purge of jalap in the morning, and repeated in a few days, with fome appearance of advantage. He was then directed to take fome pills of ſquill, foap, and rhubarb, with a draught twice a day, confifting of infuf. amar. fimp. and fal tartari. The ſkin foon became clearer and
the

the pain in his breaſt conſiderably diminiſhed. But every other circumſtance remaining the ſame, and a fluctuation in the belly being now more evident, the infuſion of Digitalis as preſcribed in caſe third, was given in the doſe of one ounce twice a day.

On the 5th day the effects were apparent, and he continued his medicine for a fortnight without nauſea, making four or five pints of water every night, but little in the day, and gradually loſing the ſymptoms of his diſeaſe.

In 1784, this perſon had a relapſe, and was again cured by ſimilar treatment.

C A S E V.

R——— H———, Aged 43. Towards the end of the year 1783, became affected with ſlight cough and expectoration of purulent matter. In December his ſkin became univerſally of a pale yellow colour. The abdomen was ſwelled and hard; his appetite little, and he complained of a violent and conſtant palpitation of the heart, which prevented him from ſleeping. The urine pale, and in ſmall quantity. The pulſe exceedingly ſtrong, and rebounding; beating 114 to 120 ſtrokes every minute. He ſuffered violent pain of his head, and was very feeble and emaciated. After bleeding, and the uſe of gentle aperient medicines, he continued to take the infuſion of Digitalis for ſome days, without any ſenſible effect. Other diuretics were tried to as little purpoſe

pose. Repeated bleeding had no effect in diminishing the violent action of the heart. He died in January following, under complicated symptoms of phthisis and ascites.

CASE VI.

A man aged 57, who had lived freely in the summer of 1784, became affected with œdematous swelling of his legs, for which he was advised to drink Fox Glove Tea. He took a four ounce bason of the infusion made strong with the green leaves, every morning for four successive days.

On the 5th he was suddenly seized with faintness and cold sweatings. I found him with a pale countenance, complaining of weakness, and of pain, with a sense of great heat in his stomach and bowels. The swelling of the legs was entirely gone, he having evacuated urine in very large quantities for the two preceding days. He was affected with frequent diarrhœa. The pulse was very quick and small, and his extremities cold.

A small quantity of broth was directed to be given him every half hour, and blisters were applied to the ancles, by which his symptoms became gradually alleviated, and he recovered perfectly in the space of three weeks; except a relapse of the anasarca, for which the Digitalis was afterwards successfully employed, in small doses, without any disagreeable consequence.

CASE

C A S E   VII.

S—— D———, a middle aged single woman, was affected in the year eighty-one, with a painful rigidity and slight inflammation of the integuments on the left side, extending from the ear to the shoulder. In every other particular she was healthy. The use of warm fomentations, and opium, with two or three doses of mercurial physic, afforded her ease and the inflammation disappeared, but was succeeded by an œdematous swelling of the part, which very gradually extended along the arm, and downward to the breast, back, and belly. Friction, electricity and mercurial ointment were amongst the number of applications unsuccessfully employed to relieve her for the space of three months, during which time she continued in good general health.

In *November* she became ascitic, passing small quantities of urine, and soon afterwards a sudden dyspnœa gave occasion to suppose an effusion of water in the thorax. The Digitalis, squills, and cantharides were given in very considerable doses without effect. She died the latter end of December following.

C A S E   VIII.

W—— C———, a collier aged 58, was attacked in the spring of 1783 with a tertian ague, which he attributed to cold, by sleeping in a coal

M   pit,

pit, and from which he recovered in a few days, except a swelling of the lower extremities, which had appeared about that time, and gradually increased for two or three months. The legs and thighs were greatly enlarged and œdematous. His belly was swelled, but no fluctuation perceptible. He made small quantities of high coloured water. The appetite bad, and pulse feeble. He had taken many medicines without relief, and was now so reduced in strength, as to sit up with difficulty. An infusion of the Digitalis was directed for him, in the proportion of one ounce of the fresh leaves to a pint of water, two ounces to be taken three times a day, until the stomach or bowels became affected. Upon the exhibition of the sixth dose, nausea supervened, and continued to oppress him at intervals for two or three days, during which he passed large quantities of pale urine. The swelling, assisted by moderate bandage rapidly diminished, and without any repetition of his medicine, at the expiration of sixteen days, he returned to his labour perfectly recovered.

O F

OF THE

PREPARATIONS and DOSES,

OF THE

FOXGLOVE.

EVERY part of the plant has more or lefs of the fame bitter tafte, varying, however, as to ftrength, and changing with the age of the plant and the feafon of the year.

ROOT.—This varies greatly with the age of the plant. When the ftem has fhot up for flower-ing, which it does the fecond year of its growth, the root becomes dry, nearly taftelefs, and inert.

Some practitioners, who have ufed the root, and been fo happy as to cure their patients without ex-citing ficknefs, have been pleafed to communicate the circumftance to me as an improvement in the ufe of the plant. I have no doubt of the truth of their remarks, and I thank them. But the cafe of Dr. Cawley puts this matter beyond difpute. The fact is, they have fortunately happened to ufe the root in its approach to its inert ftate, and confe-quently have not over dofed their patients. I could,

if

if neceſſary, bring other proof to ſhew that the root is juſt as capable as the leaves, of exciting nauſea.

STEM.—The ſtem has more taſte than the root has, in the ſeaſon the ſtem ſhoots out, and leſs taſte than the leaves. I do not know that it has been particularly ſelected for uſe.

LEAVES.—Theſe vary greatly in their efficacy at different ſeaſons of the year, and, perhaps, at different ſtages of their growth; but I am not certain that this variation keeps pace with the greater or leſſer intenſity of their bitter taſte.

Some who have been habituated to the uſe of the recent leaves, tell me, that they anſwer their purpoſe at every ſeaſon of the year; and I believe them, notwithſtanding I myſelf have found very great variations in this reſpect. The ſolution of this difficulty is obvious. They have uſed the leaves in ſuch large proportion, that the doſes have been ſufficient, or more than ſufficient, even in their moſt inefficacious ſtate. *The Leaf-ſtalks* ſeem, in their ſenſible properties, to partake of an intermediate ſtate between the leaves and the ſtem.

FLOWERS.—The petals, the chives, and the pointal have nearly the taſte of the leaves, and it has been ſuggeſted to me, by a very ſenſible and judicious friend, that it might be well to fix on the flower for internal uſe. I ſee no objection to the propoſition; but I have not tried it.

SEEDS.

S E E D S.—Thefe I believe are equally untried.

From this view of the different parts of the plant, it is fufficiently obvious why I ftill continue to pre-fer the leaves.

Thefe fhould be gathered after the flowering ftem has fhot up, and about the time that the bloffoms are coming forth.

The leaf-ftalk and mid-rib of the leaves fhould be rejected, and the remaining part fhould be dried, either in the fun-fhine, or on a tin pan or pewter difh before a fire.

If well dried, they readily rub down to a beauti-ful green powder, which weighs fomething lefs than one-fifth of the original weight of the leaves. Care muft be taken that the leaves be not fcorched in drying, and they fhould not be dried more than what is requifite to allow of their being readily re-duced to powder.

I give to adults, from one to three grains of this powder twice a day. In the reduced ftate in which phyficians generally find dropfical patients, four grains a day are fufficient. I fometimes give the powder alone ; fometimes unite it with aromatics, and fometimes form it into pills with a fufficient quantity of foap or gum ammoniac.

M 3 If

If a liquid medicine be preferred, I order a dram of these dried leaves to be infused for four hours in half a pint of boiling water, adding to the strained liquor an ounce of any spirituous water. One ounce of this infusion given twice a day, is a medium dose for an adult patient. If the patient be stronger than usual, or the symptoms very urgent, this dose may be given once in eight hours; and on the contrary in many instances half an ounce at a time will be quite sufficient. About thirty grains of the powder or eight ounces of the infusion, may generally be taken before the nausea commences.

The ingenuity of man has ever been fond of exerting itself to vary the forms and combinations of medicines. Hence we have spirituous, vinous, and acetous tinctures; extracts hard and soft, syrups with sugar or honey, &c. but the more we multiply the forms of any medicine, the longer we shall be in ascertaining its real dose. I have no lasting objection however to any of these formulæ except the extract, which, from the nature of its preparation must ever be uncertain in its effects; and a medicine whose fullest dose in substance does not exceed three grains, cannot be supposed to stand in need of condensation.

It appears from several of the cases, that when the Digitalis is disposed to purge, opium may be joined with it advantageously; and when the bowels are too tardy, jalap may be given at the same time,

without

without interfering with its diuretic effects; but I have not found benefit from any other adjunct.

From this view of the doses in which the Digitalis really ought to be exhibited, and from the evidence of many of the cases, in which it appears to have been given in quantities six, eight, ten or even twelve times more than necessary, we must admit as an inference either that this medicine is perfectly safe when given as I advise, or that the medicines in daily use are highly dangerous.

EFFECTS,

EFFECTS, RULES, and CAUTIONS.

THE Foxglove when given in very large and quickly-repeated doses, occasions sickness, vomiting, purging, giddiness, confused vision, objects appearing green or yellow; increased secretion of urine, with frequent motions to part with it, and sometimes inability to retain it; slow pulse, even as slow as 35 in a minute, cold sweats, convulsions, syncope, death.*

When given in a less violent manner, it produces most of these effects in a lower degree; and it is curious to observe, that the sickness, with a certain dose of the medicine, does not take place for many hours after its exhibition has been discontinued; that the flow of urine will often precede, sometimes accompany, frequently follow the sickness at the distance of some days, and not unfrequently be checked by it. The sickness thus excited, is extremely different from that occasioned by any other medicine; it is peculiarly distressing to the patient; it ceases, it recurs again as violent as before; and thus it will continue to recur for three or four days, at distant and more distant intervals.

These

---

* I am doubtful whether it does not sometimes excite a copious flow of saliva.—See cases at pages 115, 154, and 155.

These sufferings of the patient are generally rewarded by a return of appetite, much greater than what existed before the taking of the medicine.

But these sufferings are not at all necessary; they are the effects of our inexperience, and would in similar circumstances, more or less attend the exhibition of almost every active and powerful medicine we use.

Perhaps the reader will better understand how it ought to be given, from the following detail of my own improvement, than from precepts peremptorily delivered, and their source veiled in obscurity.

At first I thought it necessary *to bring on and continue the sickness,* in order to ensure the diuretic *effects.*

I soon learnt that the nausea being once excited, it was unnecessary to repeat the medicine, as it was certain to recur frequently, at intervals more or less distant.

Therefore my patients were ordered *to persist until the nausea came on, and then to stop.* But it soon appeared that the diuretic effects would often take place first, and sometimes be checked when the sickness or a purging supervened.

The

The direction was therefore enlarged thus—*Continue the medicine until the urine flows, or sickness or purging take place.*

I found myself safe under this regulation for two or three years ; but at length cases occurred in which the pulse would be retarded to an alarming degree, without any other preceding effect.

The directions therefore required an additional attention to the state of the pulse, and it was moreover of consequence not to repeat the doses too quickly, but to allow sufficient time for the effects of each to take place, as it was found very possible to pour in an injurious quantity of the medicine, before any of the signals for forbearance appeared.

Let the medicine therefore be given in the doses, and at the intervals mentioned above:—let it be continued until it either acts on the kidneys, the stomach, the pulse, or the bowels ; let it be stopped upon the first appearance of any one of these effects, and I will maintain that the patient will not suffer from its exhibition, nor the practitioner be disappointed in any reasonable expectation.

If it purges, it seldom succeeds well.

The patients should be enjoined to drink very freely during its operation. I mean, they should drink whatever they prefer, and in as great quantity

tity as their appetite for drink demands. This direction is the more neceffary, as they are very generally prepoffeffed with an idea of drying up a dropfy, by abftinence from liquids, and fear to add to the difeafe, by indulging their inclination to drink.

In cafes of afcites and anafarca ; when the patients are weak, and the evacuation of the water rapid ; the ufe of proper bandage is indifpenfably neceffary to their fafety.

If the water fhould not be wholly evacuated, it is beft to allow an interval of feveral days before the medicine be repeated, that food and tonics may be adminiftered ; but truth compels me to fay, that the ufual tonic medicines have in thefe cafes very often deceived my expectations.

From fome cafes which have occurred in the courfe of the prefent year, I am difpofed to believe that the Digitalis may be given in fmall dofes, viz. two or three grains a day, fo as gradually to remove a dropfy, without any other than mild diuretic effects, and without any interruption to its ufe until the cure be compleated.

If inadvertently the dofes of the Foxglove fhould be prefcribed too largely, exhibited too rapidly, or urged to too great a length ; the knowledge of a remedy to counteract its effects would be a defirable thing.

thing. Such a remedy may perhaps in time be discovered. The usual cordials and volatiles are generally rejected from the stomach; aromatics and strong bitters are longer retained; brandy will sometimes remove the sickness when only slight; I have sometimes thought small doses of opium useful, but I am more confident of the advantage from blisters. Mr. Jones (*Page* 135) in one case, found mint tea to be retained longer than other things.

CON-

CONSTITUTION of PATIENTS.

INDEPENDENT of the degree of difeafe, or of the ftrength or age of the patient, I have had occafion to remark, that there are certain conftitutions favourable, and others unfavourable to the fuccefs of the Digitalis.

From large experience, and attentive obfervation, I am pretty well enabled to decide *a priori* upon this matter, and I wifh to enable others to do the fame: but I feel myfelf hardly equal to the undertaking. The following hints, however, aiding a degree of experience in others, may lead them to accomplifh what I yet can defcribe but imperfectly.

It feldom fucceeds in men of great natural ftrength, of tenfe fibre, of warm fkin, of florid complexion, or in thofe with a tight and cordy pulfe.

If the belly in afcites be tenfe, hard, and circumfcribed, or the limbs in anafarca folid and refifting, we have but little to hope.

On the contrary, if the pulfe be feeble or intermitting, the countenance pale, the lips livid, the fkin cold, the fwollen belly foft and fluctuating, or the

the anafarcous limbs readily pitting under the preffure of the finger, we may expect the diuretic effects to follow in a kindly manner.

In cafes which foil every attempt at relief, I have
been aiming, for fome time paft, to make fuch a
change in the conftitution of the patient, as might
give a chance of fuccefs to the Digitalis.

By blood-letting, by neutral falts, by cliryftals
of tartar, fquills, and occafional purging, I have
fucceeded, though imperfectly. Next to the ufe
of the lancet, I think nothing lowers the tone of
the fyftem more effectually than the fquill, and con-
fequently it will always be proper, in fuch cafes, to
ufe the fquill ; for if that fail in its defired effect, it
is one of the beft preparatives to the adoption of the
Digitalis.

A tendency to paralytic affections, or a ftroke of
the palfy having actually taken place, is no objection to the ufe of the Digitalis ; neither does a
ftone exifting in the bladder forbid its ufe. Theo-
retical ideas of fedative effects in the former, and
apprehenfions of its excitement of the urinary organs in the latter cafe, might operate fo as to
make us with-hold relief from the patient ; but experience tells me, that fuch apprehenfions are
groundlefs.

INFER-

INFERENCES.

TO prevent any improper influence, which the above recitals of the efficacy of the medicine, aided by the novelty of the subject, may have upon the minds of the younger part of my readers, in raising their expectations to too high a pitch, I beg leave to deduce a few inferences, which I apprehend the facts will fairly support.

I. That the Digitalis will not universally act as a diuretic.

II. That it does do so more generally than any other medicine.

III. That it will often produce this effect after every other probable method has been fruitlessly tried.

IV. That if this fails, there is but little chance of any other medicine succeeding.

V. That in proper doses, and under the management now pointed out, it is mild in its operation, and gives less disturbance to the system, than squill, or almost any other active medicine.

VI. That when dropsy is attended by palsy, unsound viscera, great debility, or other complication of disease, neither the Digitalis, nor any other diuretic

retic can do more than obtain a truce to the urgency of the fymptoms; unlefs by gaining time, it may afford opportunity for other medicines to combat and fubdue the original difeafe.

VII. That the Digitalis may be ufed with advantage in every fpecies of dropfy, except the encyfted.

VIII. That it may be made fubfervient to the cure of difeafes, unconnected with dropfy.

IX. That it has a power over the motion of the heart, to a degree yet unobferved in any other medicine, and that this power may be converted to falutary ends.

PRACTICAL

PRACTICAL

REMARKS ON DROPSY,

AND SOME OTHER DISEASES.

TH E following remarks confift partly of matter of fact, and partly of opinion. The former will be permanent; the latter muft vary with the detectiou of error, or the improvement of know-ledge. I hazard them with diffidence, and hope they will be examined with candour; not by a con-traft with other opinions, but by an attentive com-parifon with the phœnomena of difeafe.

ANASARCA.

§ 1. THE anafarca is generally curable when feat-ed in the fub-cutaneous cellular membrane, or in the fubftance of the lungs.

§ 2. When the abdominal vifcera in general are greatly enlarged, which they fometimes are, with-out effufed fluid in the cavity of the abdomen; the difeafe is incurable. After death, the more folid vifcera are found very large and pale. If the ca-vity contains water, that water may be removed by diuretics.

N   § 3. In

§ 3. In swollen legs and thighs, where the resistance to pressure is considerable, the tendency to transparency in the skin not obvious, and where the alteration of posture occasions but little alteration in the state of distension, the cure cannot be effected by diuretics.

Is this difficulty of cure occasioned by spissitude in the effused fluids, by want of proper communication from cell to cell, or is the disease rather caused by a morbid growth of the solids, than by an accumulation of fluid?

Is not this disease in the limbs similar to that of the viscera (§ 2)?

§ 4. Anasarcous swellings often take place in palsied limbs, in arms as well as legs; so that the swelling does not depend merely upon position.

§ 5. Is there not cause to suspect that many dropsies originate from paralytic affections of the lymphatic absorbents? And if so, is it not probable that the Digitalis, which is so effectual in removing dropsy, may also be used advantageously in some kinds of palsy?

ASCITES,

§ 6. IF existing alone, (i. e.) without accompanying anasarca, is in children curable; in adults generally incurable by medicines. Tapping may be

used

ufed here with better chance for fuccefs than in
more complicated dropfies. Sometimes cured by
vomiting.

ASCITES and ANASARCA.

§ 7. I N C U R A B L E if dependant upon
irremediably difeafed vifcera, or on a gouty conftitution, fo debilitated, that the gouty paroxyfms no
longer continue to be formed.

In every other fituation the difeafe yields to diuretics and tonics.

ASCITES, ANASARCA, and HYDROTHORAX.

§ 8. U N D E R this complication, though the
fymptoms admit, of relief, the reftoration of the
conftitution can hardly be hoped for.

ASTHMA.

§ 9. T H E true fpafmodic afthma, a rare difeafe
—is not relieved by Digitalis.

§ 10. In the greater part of what are called
afthmatical cafes, the real difeafe is anafarca of the
lungs, and is generally to be cured by diuretics. (See
§ 1.) This is almoft always combined with fome
fwelling of the legs.

§ 11. There

§ 11. There is another kind of asthma, in which change of posture does not much affect the patient. I believe it to be caused by an infarction of the lungs. It is incurable by diuretics; but it is often accompanied with a degree of anasarca, and so far it admits of relief.

Is not this disease similar to that in the limbs at (§ 3,) and also to that of the abdominal viscera at (§ 2,)?

ASTHMA and ANASARCA.

§ 12. IF the asthma be of the kind mentioned at (§§ 9 and 11,) diuretics can only remove the accompanying anasarca. But if the affection of the breath depends also upon cellular effusion, as it mostly does, the patient may be taught to expect a recovery.

ASTHMA and ASCITES.

§ 13. A RARE combination, but not incurable if the the abdominal viscera are found. The asthma is here most probably of the anasarcous kind (§ 10;) and this being seldom confined to the lungs only, the disease generally appears in the following form.

ASTHMA,

ASTHMA, ASCITES, and ANASARCA.

§ 14. THE curability of this combination will depend upon the circumstances mentioned in the preceding section, taking also into the account the strength or weakness of the patient.

EPILEPSY.

§ 15. IN epilepsy dependant upon effusion, the Digitalis will effect a cure; and in the cases alluded to, the dropsical symptoms were unequivocal. It has not had a sufficient trial in my hands, to determine what it can do in other kinds of epilepsy.

HYDATID DROPSY

§ 16. THIS may be distinguished from common ascites, by the want of evident fluctuation. It is common to both sexes. It does not admit of a cure either by tapping or by medicine.

HYDROCEPHALUS.

§ 17. THIS disease, which has of late so much attracted the attention of the medical world, I believe, originates in inflammation; and that the water found in the ventricles of the brain after death, is the consequence, and not the cause of the illness.

It has seldom happened to me to be called upon in the earlier stages of this complaint, and the symp-

toms

toms are at firſt ſo ſimilar to thoſe uſually attendant upon dentition and worms, that it is very difficult to pronounce decidedly upon the real nature of the diſeaſe; and it is rather from the failure of the uſual modes of relief, than from any other more decided obſervation, that we at length dare to give it a name.

At firſt, the febrile ſymptoms are ſometimes ſo unſteady, that I have known them miſtaken for the ſymptoms of an intermittent, and the cure attempted by the bark.

In the more advanced ſtages, the diagnoſtics obtrude themſelves upon our notice, and put the ſituation of the patient beyond a doubt. But this does not always happen. The variations of the pulſe, ſo accurately deſcribed by thè late Dr. Whytt, do not always enſue. The dilatation of the pupils, the ſquinting, and the averſion to light, do not univerſally exiſt. The ſcreaming upon raiſing the head from the pillow or the lap, and the fluſhing of the cheeks, I once conſidered as affording indubitable marks of the diſeaſe; but in a child which I ſometime ſince attended with Dr. Aſh, the pulſe was uniformly about 85, (except during the firſt week, before we had the care of the patient.) The child never ſhewed any averſion to the light; never had dilated pupils, never ſquinted, never ſcreamed when raiſed from the lap or taken out of the bed, nor did we obſerve any remarkable fluſhing of the cheeks; and the ſleep was quiet, but ſometimes moaning.

Frequent

Frequent vomiting exifted from the firft, but ceafed for feveral days towards the conclufion. One or two worms came away during the illnefs, and it was all along difficult to purge the child. Three days before death, the right fide became flightly paralytic, and the pupil of that eye fomewhat dilated.

., After death, about two ounces and a half of water were found in the ventricles of the brain, and the veffels of the dura mater were turgid with blood.

If I am right as to the nature of hydrocephalus, that it is at firft dependant upon inflammation, or congeftion; and that the water in the ventricles is a confequence, and not a caufe of the difeafe; the curative intentions ought to be extremely different in the firft and the laft ftages.

It happens very rarely that I am called to patients at the beginning, but in two inftances wherein I was called at firft, the patients were cured by repeated topical bleedings, vomits, and purges.

Some years ago I mentioned thefe opinions, and the fuccefs of the practice refulting from them, to Dr. Quin, now phyfician at Dublin. That gentleman had lately taken his degree, and had chofen hydrocephalus for the fubject of his thefis in the year 1779. In this very ingenious effay, which he gave me the fame morning, I was much pleafed to find that the author had not only held the fame

ideas

ideas relative to the nature of the difeafe, but had alfo confirmed them by diffections.

In the year 1781, another cafe in the firft ftage demanded my attention. The reader is referred back to Cafe LXIX for the particulars.

I have not yet been able to determine whether the Digitalis can or cannot be ufed with advantage in the fecond ftage of the hydrocephalus. In Cafe XXXIII. the fymptoms of death were at hand; in Cafe LXIX. the practice, though fuccefsful, was too complicated, and in Cafe CLI. the medicine was certainly ftopped too foon.

When we confider what enormous quantities of mercury may be ufed in this complaint, without affecting the falivary glands, it feems probable that other parts may be equally infenfible to the action of their peculiar ftimuli, and therefore that the Digitalis ought to be given in much larger dofes in this, than in other difeafes.

HYDROTHORAX.

§ 18. UNDER this name I alfo include the dropfy of the pericardium.

The intermitting pulfe, and pain in the arms, fufficiently diftinguifh this difeafe from afthma, and and from anafarcous lungs.

It is very univerfally cured by the Digitalis.

§ 19. I lately

§ 19. I lately met with two cases which had been considered and treated as angina pectoris. They both appeared to me to be cases of hydrothorax. One subject was a clergyman, whose strength had been so compleatly exhausted by the continuance of the disease, and the attempts to relieve it, that he did not survive many days. The other was a lady, whose time of life made me suspect effusion. I directed her to take small doses of the pulv. Digitalis, which in eight days removed all her complaints. This happened six months ago, and she remains perfectly well.

HYDROTHORAX and ANASARCA.

§ 20. THIS combination is very frequent, and, I believe, may always be cured by the Digitalis.

§ 21. Dropsies in the chest either with or without anasarcous limbs, are much more curable than those of the belly. Probably because the abdominal viscera are more frequently diseased in the latter than in the former cases.

INSANITY.

§ 22. I APPREHEND this disease to be more frequently connected with serous effusion than has been commonly imagined.

§ 23. Where appearances of anasarca point out the true cause of the complaint, as in cases XXIV. and XXXIV.

XXXIV. the happieſt effects may be expected from the Digitalis; and men of more experience than myſelf in caſes of inſanity, will probably employ it ſuccefsfully in other leſs obvious circumſtances.

NEPHRITIS CALCULOSA.

§ 24. WE have had ſufficient evidence of the efficacy of the Foxglove in removing the Dyſuria and other ſymptoms of this diſeaſe; but probably it is not in theſe caſes preferable to the tobacco.*

OVARIUM DROPSY.

§ 25. THIS ſpecies of encyſted dropſy is not without difficulty diſtinguiſhable from an aſcites; and yet it is neceſſary to diſtinguiſh them, becauſe the two diſeaſes require different treatment and becauſe the probality of a cure is much greater in one than in the other.

§ 26. The ovarium dropſy is generally ſlow in its progreſs; for a conſiderable time the patient though ſomewhat emaciated, does not loſe the appearance of health, and the urine flows in the uſual quantity. It is ſeldom that the practitioner is called in early enough to diſtinguiſh by the feel on which ſide the cyſt originated, and the patients do not attend to that circumſtance themſelves. They generally menſtruate

---

* See an original and valuable treatiſe by **Dr. Fowler**, entitled, *Medical Reports of the Effects of Tobacco*.

ftruate regularly in the incipient ftate of the difeafe, and it is not until the preffure from the fac becomes very great, that the urinary fecretion diminifhes. In this fpecies of dropfy, the patients, upon being queftioned, acknowledge even from a pretty early date, pains in the upper and inner parts of the thighs, fimilar to thofe which women experience in a ftate of pregnancy. Thefe pains are for a length of time greater in one thigh than in the other, and I believe it will be found that the difeafe originated on that fide.

§ 27. The ovarium dropfy defies the power of medicine. It admits of relief, and fometimes of a cure, by tapping. I fubmit to the confideration of practitioners, how far we may hope to cure this difeafe by a feton or a cauftic. —— In the LXIft cafe the patient was too much reduced, and the difeafe too far advanced to allow of a cure by any method; but it teaches us that a cauftic may be ufed with fafety.

§ 28. When tapping becomes neceffary, I always advife the adoption of the waiftcoat bandage or belt, invented by the late very juftly celebrated Dr. Monro, and defcribed in the firft volume of the Medical Effays. I alfo enjoin my patients to wear this bandage afterwards, from a perfuafion that it retards the return of the difeafe. The proper ufe of bandage, when the diforder firft difcovers itfelf, certainly contributes much to prevent its increafe.

OVA-

OVARIUM DROPSY with ANASARCA.

§ 29. THE anafarca does not appear until the encyfted dropfy is very far advanced. It is then probably caufed by weaknefs and preffure. The Digitalis
removes it for a time. '

PHTHISIS PULMONALIS.

§ 30. This is a very increafing malady in the prefent day. It is no longer limited to the middle part
of life : children at five years of age die of it, and
old people at fixty or feventy. It is not confined
to the flat-chefted, the fair-fkinned, the blue eyed,
the light-haired, or the fcrophulous : it often attacks
people with full chefts, brown fkins, dark hair and
eyes, and thofe in whofe family no fcrophulous taint
can be traced. It is certainly infectious. The very
ftrict laws ftill exifting in Italy to prevent the infec-
tion from confumptive patients, were probably not
enacted originally without a fufficient caufe. We
feem to be approaching to that ftate which firft
made fuch reftrictions neceffary, and in the further
courfe of time, the difeafe will probably fall off
again, both in virulency and frequency.

§ 31. The younger part of the female fex are
liable to a difeafe very much refembling a true confumption, and from which it is difficult to diftinguifh
it ; but this difeafe is curable by fteel and bitters.
A criterion of true phthifis has been fought for in the
ftate

fiate of the teeth ; but the exceptions to that rule are numerous. An unufual dilatation of the pupil of the eye, is the moft certain characteriftic.*

§ 32. Sydenham afferts, that the bark did not more certainly cure an intermittent, than riding did a confumption. We muft not deny the truth of an affertion, from fuch authority, but we muft conclude that the difeafe was more eafily curable a century ago than it is at prefent.

§ 33. If the Digitalis is no longer ufeful in confumptive cafes, it muft be that I know not how to manage it, or that the difeafe is more fatal than formerly ; for it would be hard to deny the teftimony cited at page 9. I wifh others would undertake the enquiry.

§ 34. When phthifis is accompanied with anafarca, or when there is reafon to fufpect hydrothorax, the Digitalis will often relieve the fufferings, and prolong the life of the patient.

§ 35. Many

* Many years ago I communicated to my friend, Dr. Percival, an account of fome trials of breathing fixed air in confumptive cafes. The refults were publifhed by him in the fecond Vol. of his very ufeful Effays Medical and Experimental, and have fince been copied into other publications. I take this opportunity of acknowledging that I fufpect myfelf to have been miftaken in the nature of the difeafe there mentioned to have been cured. I believe it was a cafe of *Vomica*, and not a true *Phthifis* that was cured. The Vomica is almoft always curable. The fixed air corrects the fmell of the matter, and very fhortly removes the hectic fever. My patients not only infpire it, but I keep large jars of the effervefcing mixture conftantly at work in their chambers.

§ 35. Many years ago, during an attendance upon Mr. B———, of a confumptive family, and himfelf in the laft ftage of a phthifis; after he was fo ill as to be confined to his chamber, his breathing became fo extremely difficult and diftreffing, that he wifhed rather to die than to live, and urged me warmly to devife fome mode to relieve him. Sufpecting ferous effufion to be the caufe of this fymptom, and he being a man of fenfe and refolution, I fully explained my ideas to him, and told him what kind of operation might afford him a chance of relief; for I was then but little acquainted with the Digitalis. He was earneft for the operation to be tried, and with the affiftance of Mr. Parrott, a very refpectable furgeon of this place, I got an opening made between the ribs upon the lower and hinder part of the thorax. About a pint of fluid was immediately difcharged, and his breath became eafy. This fluid coagulated by heat.

After fome days a copious purulent difcharge iffued from the opening, his cough became lefs troublefome, his expectoration lefs copious, his appetite and ftrength returned, he got abroad, and the wound, which became very troublefome, was allowed to heal.

He then undertook a journey to London; whilft there he became worfe: returned home, and died confumptive fome weeks afterwards.

PUER-

PUERPERAL ANASARCA.

§ 36. THIS difeafe admits of an eafy and certain cure by the Digitalis.

§ 37. This fpecies of dropfy may originate from other caufes than child birth. In the beginning of laft *March*, a gentleman at Wolverhampton defired my advice for very large and painful fwelled legs and thighs. He was a temperate man, not of a dropfical habit, had great pain in his groins, and attributed his complaints to a fall from his horfe. He had taken diuretics, and the ftrongeft draftic purgatives with very little benefit. Confidering the anafarca as caufed by the difeafed inguinal glands, I ordered common poultice and mercurial ointment to the groins, three grains of pulv. fol. Digitalis night and morning, and a cooling diuretic decoction in the day-time. He foon loft his pain, and the fwellings gradually fubfided.

THE END.

MEDICAL AND PHILOSOPHICAL INTELLIGENCE

Two years ago Mr. WANT discovered the composition of a medicine which possesses the power of removing the paroxysm of Gout in a degree fully equal to the Eau Medicinale. Since that period he has had abundant experience to satisfy himself of the identity of the two medicines.

The first hint he obtained on this subject was derived from the writings of Alexander of Tralles, a Greek physician of the sixth century, whose book on Gout is one of the most valuable clinical records of antiquity, and who, in his chapter on Anodynes, remarks, that some persons take a medicine called *Dia Hermodactylum*, which produces an evacuation of watery matter from the bowels, attended with such relief from pain that patients are immediately able to walk. *But*, says he, *it has this bad property, that it disposes them who take it to be more frequently attacked with the disease.* * He speaks also of its producing nausea and loathing of food: and proceeds to describe the manner of counteracting its bad properties.—The effects here described are so similar to those resulting from the exhibition of the Eau Medicinale, that Mr. W. was led to hope that it might be the same medicine, or at least that it possessed powers of the same kind. The *Hermodactyl*, the basis of the composition, was strongly recommended by

Paulus Aegineta as a specific for gout; and such was its reputation, that we are told by Quincy it had obtained the significant name of *Anima Articulorum*—the soul of the joints. He was further encouraged to think favourably of this medicine, from its having formed a leading article in the most celebrated gout-specifics of every age. Two of these are, Turner's gout powder, and the Vienna gout decoction, the latter of which is so strongly recommended by Behrens, in the *Ephemerides Naturae Curiosorum*. It is likewise a fact notorious to every practitioner acquainted with the history of his profession, that this root has, at different periods, obtained considerable celebrity in the treatment of gout, though its general use has, after a time, been suspended; but that the occasional want of confidence in its powers arose less from its inefficiency than its misapplication, experience enables him to affirm.

The *hermodactyl* of the shops has been considered by most writers on the materia medica to be the root of the *Colchicum illyricum*; but some recorded accounts of the poisonous qualities of the *Colchicum autumnale*, and the manner in which death had been produced by it, induced Mr. W. to make his first trials with it, and his uniform success has rendered it unnecessary to make any change.

He directed a tincture to be made by infusing, for two or three days, a quantity of the fresh-sliced root of *Colchicum autumnale*, in proof spirits of wine, in the proportion of four ounces of the former to eight of the latter. This tincture he employed in all his first experiments, but as the efficacious parts of the plant are soluble in water or wine, either of these menstrua may be used; and, to produce a medicine more particularly resembling the Eau Medicinale in external circumstances, it is merely necessary to use good Sherry or Lisbon. Mr. W. purchased the root at Butler's, in Covent Garden, but it may be procured at all the physical herb shops, and under the vulgar name of *meadow saffron* may be found in every part of England.

For medicinal purposes, a recent infusion of the fresh or dried root in water is equally efficacious. Mr. W. has made extensive trials with this watery infusion, and never been disappointed in its effects. He was led to employ the dried root, from observing its variable strength when fresh, in which it appears to be much influenced by the weather and the season of the year. After rain, it contains a large quantity of water; but, on the contrary, after much sunny weather, the watery parts of the plant are evaporated, and the active qualities more condensed.

The dose of the tincture, whether it be made with water, wine, or spirit, should be the same, and should vary according to the constitution of the patient. Upon an average, we may fix two drams, or two ordinary tea-spoonfuls, as the proper quantity for an adult.

The wine of white Hellebore has been supposed by some to be the French medicine. At a very early period of the promulgation of this opinion, Mr. W. spared no pains to ascertain how far it was founded in fact. He has employed hellebore in every possible form. In some cases it appeared to be possessed of efficacy, but a series of disappointments induced him to abandon it as a medicine on which no dependence can be placed. In its mode of operation it has some properties in common with the Colchicum, or meadow saffron, but in its power of curing gout it falls infinitely short of it.

It is proper to state, that Mr. W.'s experiments have already been made in at least FORTY cases, followed by results of the most satisfactory nature, the paroxysms being always removed, and, in several instances, no return of disease having taken place after an interval of several months.

NOTES

*This case shews decidedly that a regular fit of the gout may be rapidly cured by exciting the intestines to powerful action, and that this desirable object may be accomplished by the aid of known remedies. *Vide* Tracts on Delirium Tremens, Gout, &c. by Thomas Sutton, M.D. page 206, bottom of the page.

To subdue a paroxysm of the gout, it must be observed that the operation (of cathartics) should be powerful; and, although we may not be able to show the exact reason of this, it must be kept in mind that attention to this point is the material circumstance to be relied upon for complete success in subduing the paroxysms of gout. *Idem*, p. 203, bottom of the page.

*Alston considers this to be the case. (*Vide* Alston's Materia Medica, article Hermodactylus.) But as it is very evident that the colchicum autumnale could not be the hermodactyl of Turner, as his prescription directs fifteen grains at a dose, with equal parts of other purgatives, (*vide* Allen's Synopsis Medicinae, art. Gout;) and Stoerck, who paid much attention to the operation of colchicum autumnale, states, that a quantity of less than a grain, wrapped up in crumbs of bread, and taken internally, produced alarming symptoms. A strong infusion of the linum catharticum, or purging flax, has been used by several persons in this neighbourhood, in gout, with success. This medicine produces very copious actions on the bowels.

*Of John Tomkin, Great St. Andrew-street, Seven Dials.

*De Medicamentis simplicibus et compostis.

†Hermodactyli radix et per se & ipsius decoctum habet vim purgandi: privatim arthriticis tune, cum humores defluunt exhibetur, verum stomacho nimis quam adversatur.

*Storck was a German physician of extensive reputation, the

disciple and contemporary of the great De Haen.—De Haen, in his hospital, before a numerous body of students and practitioners, tried in vain to produce the same curative results from cicuta, one of Storck's panaceas, which Storck professed to have witnessed, and challenged him publicly to demonstrate to the medical students of the university the truth of his allegations respecting it—*it was never done*. De Haen investigated the fact alleged by his former pupil respecting the cure of thirty-six cases of cancer, and found thirty of them had died the victims of the disease, and six remained uncured. See his Epistola de Cicuta.

In a contemporary publication, written by Storck of his friends, entitled "Alethophilorum quorundam Viennensum—Elucidatio necessaria Epistolae de Cicuta," De Haen's conduct was ascribed to envy; but whatever be the motive, the fact is undoubted: for the falsity of all Storck's publications on materia medica is quite proverbial.

†I am indebted to Sir Joseph Banks for a neat epigram on the colchicum, the last two lines of which are appropriate to our subject:

Illinor arthesi utiliter—soloaque podagram
At ne me *mundas* ni cupis mori.

The last idea is literally transcribed from Dioscorides.

‡I find this is copied from Dioscorides under the article Ephemerum, which he calls Colchicum. The term has probably been given to it from the supposition of its producing death *in one day*.

Geoffry, Materia Medica, vol. vi.

†"Mulieres Aegyptiae, *scribit*, multa factitant in balneis, ut pingues evadant.—Comedunt etiam adhuc multa, gallinas quippe arte pingues factas, nucemque Indicam in jure dissolutam, ac in massam redactam. Sed ex omnibus pro secreto habent singulo die, dum eunt dormitum, ad decem vulgares bulbos, pro hermodactylis a nostris Phamacopoeis receptos, quos aliqui potius Colchicum esse autumant, contostos mandere, eosque pluribus diebus, quindecim scilicet & viginti ad usque frequentant. Ex quorum usu, quod nostris mirum videbitur, nihil vel per alvum, vel vomitum, evacuant, minusque aliâ molestiâ mulieres vexantur, &c."—*De Medicinâ Aegyptiorum, Lib. III. Cap. XVI. pag.* 109.

Again:—"Mulieres pauperculae, sumptum pro aliis ferre nequeuntes, vulgares hermodactylos, quibus communiter nostri pharmacopoei utuntur, modicè contostos, aeque atque nos castaneas edimus multos unicâ vice, ad impinguescendum, devorant, ex quibus neque alvus aliquo pacto turbatur, neque aliud quippiam mali accedit. Hinc nostri pharmacopolae scire possunt, quantum, illis pro vero harmodactylo utentes, hactenus erraverint. Egoque hos non parum admiratus sum, quando Aegyptiae mulieres earum radicum (quas sine dubio si modo Dioscoridi credendum sit, Colchici esse quisque herbarum materiae peritus fatebitur) per muitos dies, ad decem & plures etiam, euntes dormitum sumpsisse, instarque castanearum comedisse, sine noxa nova, ibi saepius compererim, & c." —*Lib. IV. Cap. I.*

   **Cartheuser Materia Medica,* vol. ii.

FOR THE MEDICAL AND PHYSICAL JOURNAL.
ON MR. WANT'S DISCOVERY OF THE MODE OF PREPARING THE EAU MEDICINALE; by Dr. Sutton.

I observe in your last Number (for July), a paper written by Mr. Want on the cure of the Gout, by a medicine which he conceives to be the true eau medicinale. It certainly is a creditable effort in any gentleman to endeavour to discover of what a secret medicine, of acknowledged usefulness and powers, consists; as the public ought to have more real confidence in a medicine whose properties are known, and which the regular faculty can recommend, than in one which has not acquired such a sanction. But if it should happen that this secret medicine, whatever it may be, should be proved to possess no greater efficacy than many known remedies, then the real value of the discovery is much diminished, and it becomes a mere matter of curiosity. I consider the discovery of the composition of the French nostrum, at the present time, exactly in this point of view, because I am confident that we possess a numerous class of medicines which are as equally capable of subduing a paroxysm of gout as the eau medicinale. I much doubt, however, whether Mr. Want has arrived at the discovery of this last medicine,

214

though I am far from concluding that his paper is devoid of interest on that account; for I am fully convinced that he has announced a medicine which is capable of effecting all he has stated. The value of Mr. Want's communication, I judge, consists in announcing the cure of forty patients in the gout by a known medicine, and by exciting an action* which has been before stated to be capable of subduing the paroxysms of this disorder. It also announces the use of a drug which has not been of late employed for the purpose, if it ever was at any time; but the latter, in my opinion, is by no means so important to establish as the result of the practice. This remedy is announced by Mr. Want with a great degree of candour; and, though it may be as eligible as the eau medicinale, I judge it not to be one so generally applicable as might be wished. It may be that the drug called hermodactyl by Trallian may happen to be a very different one to that which we have used under that name;* and, as he appears to ascribe to it a more powerful cathartic operation than we find in the modern hermodactyl, Mr. Want's medicine may therefore come nearer in effect to the drug used by Trallian. But this neither proves that the colchicum autumnale is the hermodactylus of Trallian, nor that the eau medicinale is prepared from this drug. We indeed find, that he recommends scammony to be occasionally added to his medicine, in order to obtain a complete evacuation of the bowels, as may be seen by Mr. Want's quotation, which one might presume it would not need if the hermodactyl of Trallian was the real colchicum autumnale.

Several years ago I recommended a preparation of elatorium and opium to imitate the operation of the eau medicinale, and it was not only found to be equally effectual, but to operate in the same precise manner. A gentleman to whom I prescribed this medicine, in the dose of two grains to sixty drops of laudanum, and who had frequently taken the eau medicinale, told me that the sensations excited in him were precisely the same as those occasioned by the French nostrum. But the object that always seemed of the most importance to me on this subject, was not what the French medicine consisted of, so much as by what operations it produced its salutary effects. These appeared to me to be effected, in the most material and most permanent degree, by a powerful action on the bowels, although it certainly more immediately allays the violence of pain by its anodyne quality. Having come to this conclusion, if accurate, we have laid open to us a numerous class of medicines, which may effect equally beneficial purposes. This I have stated in my Tract on Gout; and I never, in curing an ordinary paroxysm of this disease in a healthy subject, think so much of the sort of purgative it is necessary to give, as of the doses which will induce the quantum of operation I wish to arrive at.

By keeping this in view, Epsom salts, aloëtic purgatives, calomel joined with other purgatives, jalap, gamboge, and other cathartics, given in such doses as to produce a powerful action on the intestines, may each accomplish all that is necessary, which, when this has been effected, may be followed by an anodyne at night; and these proceedings have caused as much benefit as I have ever heard the eau medicinale was capable of doing. The inquiry, therefore, having assumed this form, we are able to select from a large class of purgative medicines what may appear to be the most eligible for the various conditions of the disease and of constitution, and be able to attend to those idiosyncrasies that we occasionally meet with in persons under this disorder.

Thus far I can aver in the cure of gout, or an attempt to ameliorate the symptoms, that there is no state, short of that in which death appears to be quickly approaching, in which something may not be beneficially done by a prudent use of purgatives, and by having the whole class of them thrown open for selection. But if, on the contrary, the proper virtues of purgatives for the cure of gout can only be supposed to reside in such as the French medicine, or in such drugs as the colchicum autumnale, or as the elaterium, or as hellebore, then we should find numerous instances in which we would rather allow nature to take her course, than endeavour to controul the gout by medicines which might promote a very powerful effect on feeble constitutions, on irritable stomachs, and on other conditions in respect to age, disease, habit, &c.

By the proper use of purgative medicines in numerous instances of gout, I have seen the paroxysms of this disease overcome in the short space of a few hours, and the entire restoration of the limb affected to follow in a few days: in others, where all this benefit could not be expected to ensue, I have observed the pain to be quickly subdued, and the patient to return to a better state of limbs than before the attack of the disease. In only one instance have I found the powers of purgatives to subdue a paroxysm of gout, and a perfect restoration not to follow, where it might have been expected. This case was also as little benefitted by the eau medicinale. The patient had, however, the satisfaction to find an increase of healthful feelings, by pursuing the plan laid down in my Tract on Gout, though the paroxysms, although ameliorated, continued to return. It is too early yet to judge how far the plan laid down for this patient may be wanting in ultimate success. We ought not, however, to be discouraged by a few cases not suffering all the controul that appears to be capable of being effected in a great majority; nor ought those to detract much from the important views in which the cure of gout has of late years been placed; nor should the benefit capable of being attained by many be disregarded, because it cannot be extended to all. In the case alluded to, there are circumstances which evidently separate it from the ordinary and concurring symptoms of the gout, though, on a superficial view of the disease, it would be difficult to consider it to belong to any other species of disorder.

THOMAS SUTTON, M.D.

Croom's Hill, Greenwich,
    July 4, 1814.

MR. WANT *in answer to* DR. SUTTON.

The preceding observations are made with a view to depreciate my discovery of the mode of preparing the Eau Medicinale, because, as Dr. Sutton says, he is confident we possess a numerous class of remedies which are as capable of subduing a paroxysm of gout as the eau medicinale. Were this assertion supported by the experience of the profession, my discovery would, I admit, be of no value. If salts, magnesia, and rhubarb, will cure gout, as Dr. S. would have us believe, there can be no necessity for having recourse to a potent and deleterious drug, as mine is. But I can affirm, from repeated experiment, that no one of this numerous class of remedies deserves the character bestowed upon them. The doctor may be very correct when he says that Epsom salts and aloes have done every thing *he has heard* the eau medicinale is capable of doing; for, to adopt his own language, if it should *happen to be* that he is proved to be totally unacquainted with the curative properties, or the sensible effects of that remedy, the efficacy of these medicines may not be much overrated.

The infallibility of this class of medicines is maintained throughout the whole paper, but the sentiment is so diffused that it is difficult to fix upon a sentence sufficiently decisive to afford matter fit for quotation. The author, indeed, in one place distinctly asserts that there is no state short of that in which death is actually approaching, in which something may not beneficially be done by the prudent use of purgatives; and such has been the success of his practice, that in only one instance has he found the powers of purging to subdue a paroxysm of gout without a perfect restoration following; and he never thinks so much of the *kind* of purgative, as of the *quantum* of operation necessary to be induced. After having established that *all purgatives* will cure gout, the doctor proceeds to show that my medicine operates by exciting an action (on the bowels) which had before been stated to be capable of curing the disease. Now, the legitimate inference from these premises would be, that, although I did not deserve to be immortalized for the discovery, yet my medicine, being a purgative, was at least capable of curing the gout. But Dr. S. draws a very different conclusion, for although, he observes, the medicine may be equally eligible with the eau medicinale, yet he judges it not to be so extensively applicable as might be wished. Let it, however, be understood, that I quarrel with this conclusion only, as being inconsistent with what the author had previously maintained as indisputable facts, for it requires no peculiar sagacity to discover that this or any other known remedy is not so universally applicable as might be wished. I have made no promises of infallibility; I simply state that this medicine does that which the eau medicinale is capable of performing; and I recommend it to those only who have experienced the good effects of that remedy.

That it is not so extensively applicable as could be wished, may be collected from my own paper, wherein I have expressly adverted to its bad properties. I have there stated, that in some instances its employment may be attended with consequences fatal to the patient, particularly when administered without regard to the peculiar circumstances of the case. That this expression implies the existence of a case in which it is inapplicable, is a proposition that surely cannot be denied.

The assertion that all purgatives will cure gout, is so obviously unsupported by common experience, that our readers will scarcely require its refutation; and it only remains for me to show, that the curative powers of the colchicum autumnale are quite unconnected with its purgative operation. Upon this I may observe, that in many cases it removes the paroxysm of gout without *any* *sensible operation of any kind.* This fact is *very notorious.* If Dr. S. requires the proof of it, I may instance (among many others) the case of the illustrious President of the Royal Society, long known to have been a martyr to the disease. Sir Joseph Banks assures me, that in him the eau medicinale never produces any action on the bowels, while it never fails to relieve him; and he farther states, that the accidental occurrence of purging will generally bring on a fit of the gout, and, if present, materially aggravate the complaint. But this seems to arise from a peculiarity of constitution not constantly met with; though we are not without other examples of the same kind. It was probably the same idiosyncracy which induced Sydenham so strongly to deprecate the employment of purgatives under any circumstances in gout. Lucian, in his poetical and very accurate account of this disease, intimates the tendency of purging to produce or aggravate the fit, when he makes the goddess Podagra say, she would fall with greater fury upon those who purged themselves with the hiera picra. These instances, however, have not made me insensible to the value of that class of remedies, for, in the month of August 1811, I wrote an essay for the Med. and Phys. Journal expressly for the purpose of recommending them, *not as infallible*, but as being most extensively useful. The elaterium, which Dr. S. takes to himself the credit of introducing into practice, though his Tract did not appear till the year 1813, was first recommended by *me* in 1811, accompanied with cases of success from its employment, and it may be remarked that one case is there related where it failed,* as purgatives frequently do; and the patient has since my discovery been invariably relieved, and the paroxysm removed, by the colchicum.

It cannot be denied, as *I have shown in my former essay*, that the drastic purgatives, (the foremost among which is elaterium,) are, if properly administered, very useful in the treatment of this complaint; but they have failed, and will fail in a multitude of cases, perfectly within the influence of the meadow saffron.

Dr. Sutton says, the hermodactyl described by Trallian *may happen to be* a very different medicine from that which we use under that name. If it *only may happen to be*, it *may not be*, different. If the doctor had any doubts respecting it, it was incumbent upon him to state the reasons which induced him to differ. He assumes indeed that Alexander ascribed to the hermodactyl a more powerfully purgative operation that we find in the modern hermodactyl. I am at a loss to conceive what foundation there can be for this opinion, when we are expressly told by this author, as Dr. S. unaccountably admits, that even in cases where a large dose of his medicine seems to have been prescribed, if a fuller evacuation from the bowels was desirable, scammony was to be added.

Here appears no evidence of extraordinary purgative powers possessed by the hermodactyl, and, admitting that it sometimes occasioned the watery evacuation from the bowels described in my last, yet we are led to conclude there were cases where it failed to produce this effect, and where the addition of stronger purgatives was rendered necessary. It cannot escape notice that from a part of this quotation (   ) it appears that even the addition of so much scammony (16 grains) was supposed to render it but a *mild purge*. In my experiments with the eau medicinale, colchicum, and the modern imported hermodactyl, I find they are also severally very variable, and equally uncertain in their operation, which seems to be governed by constitutional peculiarity, so much so that in scarcely two persons have they precisely the same effect. This fact has been universally remarked with respect to the Eau Medicinale; and it is so striking in the other two as to add, in my opinion, very considerably to the evidence of their identity. In the case of Mr. Wallis, of Judd-street, now under my care, a full dose of the Tincture of Colchicum produced a sickness with vomiting, which continued to harass him for twenty-four hours, and yet this extreme dose produced no purgative operation whatever. I have witnessed the same effect so frequently, that I have no hesitation in maintaining, that in a multitude of cases, if given in a dose just sufficient to cure the patient, and no more, it will be found to exert no purgative quality whatever, and very little sensible operation of any kind. This has probably been observed by those writers on the materia medica who affirm that the modern hermodactyl has scarcely any purgative power, and who, from an erroneous idea of the stronger purgative qualities of the ancient medicine, are from this circumstance induced to believe them essentially different. But, if we extend our researches, even among the ancients we shall find the same virtue and the same power ascribed to their hermodactyl. In the compositions of the Arabian writer, Mesue,* it is generally, if not invariably, mixed up with drastic purgatives, which generally constitute the greater bulk of the compound. Dr. S. refers to Alston, in support of his opinion; but this writer has furnished us with a striking quotation from Mesue, which refutes himself. The Arabian physician tells us, in the most unequivocal terms, that the hermodactyl, (the ancient,) *if unmixed with other medicines, is scarcely a purgative:*—"per se enim tarde et imbecille vacuat." Paulus Aegineta, who is said to have practiced about fifty years after Trallian, tells us the hermodactyl moves the bowels, but does not lead us to expect strong purgative effects from it.†

Thus we find the same degree of power ascribed to both the modern and ancient drug by the writers of their respective times; and, if we attentively investigate the subject, we shall discover also the same contradictions and the same implications of the uncertainty of their operation, which I have discovered to be equally characteristic of the meadow saffrom and the eau medicinale. There seems then no reason to believe them to be different medicines, from the supposed discrepancy between the modern and ancient writers.

Impressed with the belief, that the modern hermodactyl possesses less purgative powers than that described by the ancients, Dr. S. conjectures that the colchicum autumnale, on account of its stronger operation, may more nearly resemble the drug prescribed by Trallian. That it does not only resemble Trallian's drug, but is the same medicine, is a fact of which I do not entertain the smallest doubt; but I do not discover this resemblance in the stronger purgative operation it is supposed to be enbued with. I have before denied that there is any foundation for believing this strong purgative power to be an *invariable* property of the ancient hermodactyl, from which, if correct, it will follow that this supposition of our author is entirely gratuitous. In the case of Mr. Wallis, before adverted to, it had no such operation, though given in an *extreme dose*. Upon what authority, I would ask, does the doctor suppose this plant to be possessed of that quality? Certainly not from his own personal observation, or we should never have had the account of Storck's experiment upon himself,* brought as an evidence on the occasion, a story more ridiculous and monstrous than any to be found in Baron Munchausen, and which can only be equalled by the countless falsehoods contained in his several publications.

The writers on the materia medica are generally silent as to this purgative effect of colchicum.† The English dispensatories who quote from Storck never hint at it. I have not time at present to peruse Storck's book, (which I have never yet thought of sufficient importance to procure, on account of his notorious inaccuracies;) but it is reasonable to suppose, that if he had seen it exert a purgative operation, he would have named it, and they would have copied him. I am not acquainted with any writer who has himself seen this effect; but the little time allowed to an answer of this kind in a public Journal, will not permit me to enquire very minutely into the circumstance. Dioscorides, as well as some modern authors, are of one accord as to its poisonous qualities. The

former of these says, the colchicum, if *eaten*, like
the fungi, kills by strangulation, but never mentions purging.

Geoffry, who seems to be unacquainted with
the properties of the plant from personal observation, says, "it is related that those who *eat it*
experience itchings throughout the whole body,
tearing pains in the bowels, with heat and weight
in the stomach. As the symptoms increase, blood
is voided by stool, and the colchicum comes away
in pieces."‡ I have seen cases in which it produced
a most alarming sense of suffocation, from the
globulus hystericus and flatulent distension of
the abdomen, without purging. Though more
commonly, in a full dose, it has this effect; which
if it does take place, immediately removes the
sense of suffocation. This is one of the circumstances in which I have observed, as referred to in
my last, such coincidence in effect between the
hellebore (which rarely purges) and this
medicine.

One author only, Ludovicus, relates, that a
single root of colchicum almost killed a patient *by
purging*. Garidel, in his Histoire des Plantes des
environs d'Aix, records, that a servant whom he
attended was killed by taking the flowers for an
intermitting fever, in which it is said to be useful.
The symptoms were probably those mentioned
above, which he terms "anxietés et des tranchés
pendant trois jours;" no purging is mentioned.
The Turks are said to intoxicate themselves with
the flowers macerated in wine.*

Prosper Alpinus says the colchicum is perfectly
inert, and that the Aegytian women fatten themselves with the *roasted* roots, often eating twenty
in the course of the day, without any evacuation

from the stomach or bowels.† But let it be observed, these roots were *roasted*, the process of which may materially alter their properties. Thus the onion, an acrid, stimulating, pungent root, when roasted loses all these qualities, and the same is true of many other plants that could be named.

Cartheuser, misled by this quotation, says, that the plant growing near him *also* has neither diuretic or cathartic power, nor does it possess any noxious property.—"*Id compertum habco* nostri pariter colchici communis, in Marchia et Silesia superiori crescentes radices nec *catharsin nec largiorem diuresin* concitari nec hominibus etiam lethiferas et saltem noxias existere."*

A difference of soil and climate *might* produce a variation in the strength of this drug, but it will be easy to account for the contradictory statements of authors respecting it by the singular diversity of its operation in different constitutions. The opinions of Alpinus may be clearly traced to the fact of his colchicum having been roasted, and others (*caeci cacos sequentes*) have copied him without taking the pains to inquire whether he was right or wrong. Its history is one of the most striking instances of the careless manner in which medical investigations are for the most part carried on. Here is a plant possessing peculiar powers,and is described as far back as the time of Dioscorides, and by most, if not all, succeeding writers on materia medica; and yet these properties have invariably escaped observation by those whose business, as authors, it ought to have been to have ascertained its effects.

The identity of the tincture of colchicum and eau medicinale, is a question which can only be determined by attentive examination, and comparison of their respective operations on the human body. I will pledge my professional reputation for the truth of what I have alledged on this subject. My practice in gout has been very great, and, where these remedies appeared likely to be useful, I have administered them with the most careful observation of their effect, and have never once entertained a doubt of their being the same medicines. I am assisted in forming my judgment by the testimony of those who have taken both medicines. I have had intercourse with many of the most distinguished literary characters of this kingdom, who are conversant both with the appearance and properties of the French remedy; and they are *unanimous* in expressing their convictions that the two compositions are identically the same. When considering the question of identity, it may be useful to advert to the fact that one Wedelius, a continental physician, sold an empirical preparation of colchicum, which, like the French nostrum, was extolled as a panacea. This, indeed, is so very common with advertized medicines, that I should not think the circumstance worth notice, if the catalogue of its virtues did not bear some resemblance to that which we find in Husson's original advertisement. It is also deserving of remark, that the account of this nostrum is contained in a System of Materia Medica (by Geoffry) well known in France, where Husson lived.

In the hurry of drawing up this answer, I may have possibly omitted some particulars important to have been mentioned. Should this hereafter appear to be the case, I shall willingly resume the subject: at present I shall merely add, that my convictions respecting these medicines are unalterably fixed.

JOHN WANT,
Surgeon to the Northern Dispensory.

No. 9, *North Crescent,*
Bedford-square.

ON THE USE OF NITRITE OF AMYL IN ANGINA PECTORIS*

BY T. LAUDER BRUNTON B.Sc., M.B.

Reprinted from: Lancet 2:97-98, 1867

Few things are more distressing to a physician than to stand beside a suffering patient who is anxiously looking to him for that relief from pain which he feels himself utterly unable to afford. His sympathy for the sufferer, and the regret he feels for the impotence of his art, engrave the picture indelibly on his mind, and serve as a constant and urgent stimulus in his search after the causes of the pain, and the means by which it may be alleviated.

Perhaps there is no class of cases in which such occurrences as this take place so frequently as in some kinds of cardiac disease, in which angina pectoris forms at once the most prominent and the most painful and distressing symptom. This painful affection is defined by Dr. Walshe as a paroxysmal neurosis, in which the heart is essentially concerned, and the cases included in this definition may be divided into two classes.

In the first and most typical there is severe pain in the precordial region, often shooting up the neck and down the arms, accompanied by dyspnoea and a most distressing sense of impending dissolution. The occurrence and departure of the attack are both equally sudden, and its duration is only a few minutes.

In the second class, which from its greater frequency is probably the more important, though the pain and dyspnoea may both be very great, the occurrence of the attack is sometimes gradual, and its departure generally so; its duration is from a few minutes to an hour and a half or more, and the sense of impending dissolution is less marked or altogether absent.

Brandy, ether, chloroform, ammonia, and other stimulants have hitherto been chiefly relied upon for the relief of angina pectoris; but the alleviation which they produce is but slight, and the duration of the attack is but little affected by them.

In now publishing a statement of the results which I have obtained in the treatment of angina pectoris by nitrite of amyl, I have to observe that the cases in which I employed this remarkable substance belonged rather to the second than the first of the classes above described.

Nitrite of amyl was discovered by Balard; and further investigated by Guthrie,* who noticed its property of causing flushing of the face, throbbing of the carotids, and acceleration of the heart's action, and proposed it as a resuscitative in drowning, suffocation, and protracted fainting.

Little attention, however, was paid to it for some years, till it was again taken up by Dr. B. W. Richardson, who found that it caused paralysis of the nerves from the periphery inwards, diminished the contractility of muscles, and caused dilatation of the capillaries, as seen in the web of the frog's foot.

Dr. Arthur Gamgee, in an unpublished series of experiments both with the sphygmograph and haemadynometer, has found that it greatly lessened the arterial tension both in animals and man; and it was these experiments—some of which I was fortunate enough to witness—which led me to try it in angina pectoris.

During the past winter there has been in the clinical wards one case in which the anginal pain was very severe, lasted from an hour to an hour and a half, and recurred every night, generally between two and four A.M.; besides several others in whom the affection, though present, was less frequent and less severe. Digitalis, aconite, and lobelia inflata were given in the intervals, without producing any benefit; and brandy and other diffusible stimulants during the fit produced little or no relief. When chloroform was given so as to produce partial stupefaction, it relieved the pain for the time; but whenever the senses again became clear, the pain was as bad as before. Small bleedings of three or four ounces, whether by cupping or venesection, were, however, always beneficial; the pain being completely absent for one night after the operation, but generally returning on the second. As I believed the relief produced by the bleeding to be due to the diminution it occasioned in the arterial tension, it occurred to me that a substance which possesses the power of lessening it in such an eminent degree as nitrite of amyl would probably produce the same effect, and might be repeated as often as necessary without detriment to the patient's health. On application to my friend Dr. Gangee, he kindly furnished me with a supply of pure nitrite which he himself had made; and on proceeding to try it in the wards, with the sanction of the visiting physician, Dr. J. Hughes Bennett, my hopes were completely fulfilled. On pouring from five to ten drops of the nitrite on a cloth and giving it to the patient to inhale, the physiological action took place in from thirty to sixty seconds; and simultaneously with the flushing of the face the pain completely disappeared, and generally did not return till its wonted time next night. Occasionally it began to return about five minutes after its first disappearance; but on giving a few drops more it again disappeared, and did not return. On a few occasions I have found that while the pain disappeared from every other part of the chest, it remained persistent at a spot about two inches to the inside of the right nipple, and the action of the remedy had to be kept up for several minutes before this completely subsided. In almost all other cases in which I have given it, as well as in those in which it has been tried by my friends, the pain has at once completely disappeared. In cases of aneurism, where the pain was constant, inhalation of the nitrite gave no relief, but where it was spasmodic or subject to occasional exacerbations it either completely removed or greatly relieved it. It may be as well to note that in those cases in which it failed, small bleedings were likewise useless.

From observations during the attack, and from an examination of numerous sphygmographic tracings taken while the patients were free from pain, while it was coming on, at its height, passing off under the influence of amyl, and again completely gone, I find that when the attack comes on gradually the pulse becomes smaller, and the arterial tension greater as the pain increases in severity. During the attack the breathing is quick, the pulse small and rapid, and the arterial tension high: owing, I believe, to contraction of the systemic capillaries. As the nitrite is inhaled the pulse becomes slower and fuller, the tension diminished, and the breathing less hurried. On those occasions when the pain returned after an interval of a few minutes, the pulse, though showing small tension, remained small in volume, and not till the volume as well as tension of the pulse became normal, did I feel sure that the pain would not return.

As patients who suffer from angina are apt to become plethoric, and greater relaxation of the vessels is then required before the tension is sufficiently lowered, I think it is advisable to take away a few ounces of blood every few weeks. When the remedy is used for a long time, the dose requires to be increased before the effect is produced. A less quantity is sufficient when it is used with a cone of blotting-paper, as recommended by Dr. Richardson, than when it is poured on a large cloth. From its power of paralysing both nerves and muscles, Dr. Richardson thinks it may prove useful in tetanus; and I believe that, by relaxing the spasm of the bronchial tubes, it might be very beneficial in spasmodic asthma. I have tried it in a case of epilepsy, but the duration of the fit seemed little affected by it. It produces relief in some kinds of headache, and in one of neuralgia of the scalp it relieved the severe shooting pain, though an aching feeling still remained.

While cholera was present in Edinburgh during last autumn, Dr. Gangee proposed it as a remedy during the stage of collapse, a condition in which there are good grounds for supposing that the small arteries, both systemic and pulmonic, are in a state of great contraction. No well-marked case afterwards occurring in the town, he was deprived of an opportunity of putting it to the test, but it is a medicine well worthy of a trial, and should another epidemic unhappily occur it may prove our most valuable remedy.

Edinburgh, July, 1867.

NOTES

*Lancet 2: 97-98, 1867
*Journal of the Chemical Society, 1859.

NITRO-GLYCERINE AS A REMEDY FOR ANGINA PECTORIS.

By WILLIAM MURRELL, M.R.C.P.,

Some twenty years ago a controversy took place in the pages of the *Medical Times and Gazette,* on the properties, physiological and therapeutical, of the substance known to chemists as nitro-glycerine. The discussion was opened by Mr. A. G. Field, then of Brighton, who described in detail the symptoms he had experienced from taking two drops of a one per cent solution of nitro-glycerine in alcohol. About three minutes after the dose had been placed on his tongue he noticed a sensation of fulness in both sides of the neck, succeeded by nausea. For a moment or two there was a little mental confusion, accompanied by a loud rushing noise in the ears, like steam passing out of a tea-kettle. He experienced a feeling of constriction around the lower part of the neck, his forehead was wet with perspiration, and he yawned frequently. These sensations were succeeded by slight headache and a dull, heavy pain in the stomach, with a decided feeling of sickness, though without any apprehension that it would amount to vomiting. He felt languid and

disinclined for exertion, either mental or physical. This condition lasted for half an hour, with the
exception of the headache, which continued till
the next morning. These symptoms Mr. Field
describes as resulting from a single dose of one-
fiftieth of a grain. Thinking that possibly he
might be unusually susceptible to the action of the
drug, he induced a friend to take a dose. The
gentleman experienced such decided effects
from merely touching his tongue with the cork of
the bottle containing the nitro-glycerine solution
that he refused to have anything more to do with
it. A lady suffering from toothache, on whose
tongue Mr. Field placed about half a drop of the
same solution, experienced a pulsation in the
neck, fulness in the head, throbbing in the temples, and slight nausea. The toothache subsided
and she became partly insensible, disliking much
to be roused. When fully sensible she had a
headache, but the toothache was gone. Another
of Mr. Field's patients, a stout, healthy young
woman, accidentally swallowed a small piece of
lint dipped in the nitro-glycerine, whilst being
applied to a decayed tooth. In about five minutes,
after feeling giddy and sick, with headache, she
became insensible. Her countenance, naturally
florid, was unaltered, breathing tranquil, pulse
full, and rather quickened. She recovered in
about three minutes, after the administration of a
stimulant. Some headache was complained of,
but the toothache was gone. Mr. Field, in conclusion, offered some suggestions as to the
therapeutical uses of the drug, and stated that he
had not met with a single well-defined case of
neuralgia or spasmodic disease in which it had
failed to afford some relief.

This paper was followed by a letter from Dr. Thorowgood, in the main confirmatory of Mr. Field's observations. He, after taking a small dose, experienced "a tensive headache over the eyes and nose, extending also behind the ears, and soon followed by a tight, choking feeling about the throat, like strangulation. Neither loss of consciousness nor nausea was experienced, and a walk by the sea soon did away with the unpleasant feeling."

These statements did not long remain unchallenged, their accuracy being called in question by Dr. George Harley, of University College, and Dr. Fuller, of St. George's. Dr. Harley, having obtained some nitro-glycerine of the same strength as Mr. Field's, commenced his observations by touching his tongue with the cork of the bottle containing the solution. He experienced "a kind of sweet and burning sensation, and soon after a sense of fulness in the head, and slight tightness about the throat, without, however, any nausea or faintness." After waiting a minute or two these effects went off, and Dr. Harley was inclined to think "they were partially due to imagination." Determined, however, as he says, to give the drug a fair chance, he swallowed five drops more, and as this did not cause any increased uneasiness, he took, in the course of a few minutes, another ten drops of the solution. Being at the time alone, he became alarmed lest he should have taken an over-dose, and very soon his pulse rose to above 100 in a minute. The fulness in the head and constriction in the throat were, he thought, more marked than after the smaller dose. In a minute or two the pulse fell to 90, but the fulness in the head lasted some time, and was followed by a slight headache. To two medical friends Dr. Harley administered respectively twenty-eight and thirty-eight drops in divided doses without the production of any symptoms. Some pure nitro-glycerine was then obtained, and of this Dr. Harley took, in the course of a few minutes, a drop, equivalent to a hundred drops of the solution previously employed. The only symptoms produced were a quickened pulse, fulness in the head, and some tightness in the throat; but as these passed off in a few minutes, Dr. Harley considered that they were probably the effects of "fear and imagination." On a subsequent occasion he took, in the course of three-quarters of an hour, a quantity of the nitroglycerine solution equivalent to 199½ drops of the solution used by Mr. Field, with the production of no more disagreeable symptoms than those he had experienced in his former trials. The quickening of the heart's action he ascribed to fear, but the head and neck sensations were, he considered, "too constant to be attributed to the same cause," although he thought they were exaggerated by the imagination. Dr. Harley, in conclusion, states that he experimented on ten different gentlemen with nitro-glycerine solution, obtained from four different sources, without witnessing any dangerous effects when administered in the above doses; but he adds that, if taken pure, great caution should be used.

Dr. Fuller, whose observations were made in conjunction with Dr. Harley, commenced by taking two drops of a one per cent solution. In the course of a minute he felt, or "fancied he felt," some fulness in the head, but was not conscious of any other unusual sensation. A little later he took one-sixth of a drop of pure nitro-glycerine, equivalent to about seventeen drops of the solution spoken of by Mr. Field. Two minutes later his pulse had risen to 96, and there was an increased fulness about the head, but without giddiness or confusion of thought. The pupils were not affected, and he did not experience any unusual sensation beyond that already mentioned. A quarter of an hour later he took a dose equal to $33^2 1/3$ drops of Mr. Field's solution, and a few minutes later another dose equivalent to 50 drops. He felt somewhat nervous, and for a few minutes the surface of the body was covered with a clammy perspiration; his pulse intermitted occasionally, and he experienced an increase of fulness about the head. Whether the acceleration of the pulse observed in the first instance was attributable to the effects of the drug he was unable to decide, but his own impression was that it was merely the result of nervousness and excitement; for, had it been otherwise, it is not likely, he says, "that the pulse would have fallen to its natural standard within so short a period after taking the larger doses." The fulness in the head might, he considered, have been attributed in part to the same cause, but a sense of discomfort in the head lasting some hours was, he thought, really due to the drug. As the result of these observations, Dr. Fuller concluded that nitro-glycerine was incapable of producing the effects that had been ascribed to it, and that it might be taken with impunity in considerable quantity.

In a second communication to the same journal Mr. Field reasserted the correctness of his observations, and maintained that a reasonable explanation of the very different results obtained by different observers might be found in the great variation in strength to which the drug is liable. He considered, too, that the conditions under which the drug was taken had much to do with its action. When the system is worn out by fatigue, he says, it is more likely to act powerfully than when taken under less unfavourable conditions. On the occasion of taking the dose which produced in him such startling effects, his nervous energy had been impaired by an unusually hard day's work. He found that under more favourable conditions he could take the same dose with the production of nothing worse than headache. Having in his experiments on himself experienced the greatest variation in the strength of different specimens of nitro-glycerine, he was disposed to think, on reading the account given by Dr. Fuller and Dr. Harley, that they had used a less powerful agent. He accordingly called on Dr. Fuller, and induced him to take a dose of the solution he had used, but, to his surprise, he experienced little beyond headache. On the same day Mr. Field administered to a hospital patient suffering from hemicrania two drops of the solution. In about a minute he became pallid, felt sick and giddy, his forehead was covered with perspiration, and he sank on the bed by which he was standing almost unconscious, his pulse failing so as scarcely to be felt. After the administration of a little ammonia the circulation became more vigorous, and in twenty minutes there was a marked diminution of the pain, and he experienced a great desire to sleep, a luxury of which his sufferings had almost deprived him on previous nights. Mr. Field administered small doses of the drug to several other people, all of whom were distinctly affected by it.

Mr. Field's observations respecting the activity of the drug were also confirmed by Mr. F. Augustus James, a student of University College. He took a single drop of the one per cent solution. In the course of a few minutes he experienced a sensation as if he were intoxicated. This was quickly followed by a dull aching pain at the back of the head, which was alternately better and worse, each accession becoming more and more severe. It soon extended to the forehead and the back of the neck, in which there was a decided feeling of stiffness. He also experienced some difficulty of deglutition, succeeded by nausea, retching, and flatulence. A profuse perspiration ensued, and in a quarter of an hour the symptoms began to abate, but he continued dull and heavy. His pulse, he found, had risen from 80 to 100. Considerable headache remained, which increased in the after part of the day, so that at six o'clock he was compelled to go to bed. At break of day he was not relieved, but after a few hours' more sleep he felt quite well again.

Mr. G. S. Brady, of Sutherland, obtained very decided results from the administration of large doses of nitro-glycerine to a lady suffering from severe facial neuralgia. He gave two minims and a half of Morson's five per cent solution in a little water. In the course of two or three minutes she began to complain of sickness and faintness; these rapidly increased; there was for a few minutes unconsciousness accompanied by convulsive action of the muscles of the face, and stertorous breathing. After swallowing some

brandy-and-water, she vomited, and the unpleasant symptoms gradually subsided. Mr. Brady also
mentions the case of a relative of his, a chemist,
who took a drop of the five per cent solution in
water. Shortly afterwards a feeling of sickness
and pain at the epigastrium came on, and he left
his desk to pace about the shop,thinking to walk
off the uncomfortable sensations. Instead of this,
they grew worse, and an intolerable sense of oppression and swimming in the head, with spasmodic twitching of the limbs, supervened. He
had barely time to call his assistant when he fell
back insensible. Cold water was freely dashed
over the face, and the unconsciousness soon passed away. No vomiting ensued, but the sensation
of sickness lasted for some time.

Being greatly interested in this curious controversy, and being quite at a loss to reconcile the
conflicting statements of the different observers,
or arrive at any conclusion respecting the properties of the drug, I determined to try its action on
myself. Accordingly I obtained some one per cent
solution. One afternoon, whilst seeing out-pa-
tients, I remembered that I had the bottle in my
pocket. Wishing to taste it, I applied the mois-
tened cork to my tongue, and a moment after, a
patient coming in, I had forgotten all about it.
Not for long, however, for I had not asked my
patient half a dozen questions before I experienced a violent pulsation in my head, and Mr. Field's
observations rose considerably in my estimation.
The pulsation rapidly increased, and soon became so severe that each beat of the heart seemed
to shake my whole body. I regretted that I had not
taken a more opportune moment of trying my
experiments, and was afraid the patient would

notice my distress, and think that I was either ill or intoxicated. I was quite unable to continue my questions, and it was as much as I could do to tell him to go behind the screen and undress, so that his chest might be examined. Being temporarily free from observation, I took my pulse, and found that it was much fuller than natural, and considerably over 100. The pulsation was tremendous, and I could feel the beating to the very tips of my fingers. The pen I was holding was violently jerked with every beat of the heart. There was a most distressing sensation of fullness all over the body, and I felt as if I had been running violently. I remained quite quiet for four or five minutes, and the most distressing symptoms gradually subsided. I then rose to examine the patient, but the exertion of walking across the room intensified the pulsation. I hardly felt steady enough to perform percussion, and determined to confine my attention to auscultation. The act of bending down to listen caused such an intense beating in my head that it was almost unbearable, and each beat of the heart seemed to me to shake not only my head, but the patient's body too. On resuming my seat I felt better, and was soon able to go on with my work, though a splitting headache remained for the whole afternoon. Were my symptoms due to nervousness or anxiety? Certainly not. I will not say that I discredited Mr. Field's observations, but after Dr. Harley's positive assertions I certainly did not expect to obtain any very definite results from so small a dose. Moreover, at the moment of the onset of the symptoms I was engaged in the consideration of another subject, and had forgotten all about the nitro-glycerine. I did nothing to intensify the symptoms, but, on the contrary, should have been only too glad to have got rid of them. The headache, I can most positively affirm, was anything but fancy. Since then I have taken the drug some thirty or forty times, but I never care to do so unless I am quite sure that I can sit down and remain quiet for a time, if necessary. It uniformly produces in me the same symptoms, but they are comparatively slight if I refrain from moving about or exertion of any kind. The acceleration of the pulse is very constant, although sometimes it amounts to not more than ten beats in the minute. The temperature remains unaffected. The pulsation is often so severe as to be acutely painful. It jerks the whole body so that a book held in the hand is seen to move quite distinctly at each beat of the heart. The amount of pulsation may be roughly measured by holding a looking-glass in the hand and throwing the reflection into a dark corner of the room. Before taking the drug the bright spot may be kept steady, but as soon as the pulsation begins it is jerked violently from side to side. I have taken all doses from one minim to ten, sometimes simply dropped on the tongue, at others swallowed on sugar or in water. I have not ventured to take more than fifteen minims in a quarter of an hour. Once or twice a ten-minim dose has produced less pulsation than I have experienced at other times from a single drop; but then with the larger quantity one is careful to avoid even the slightest movement. After a five-minim dose I usually experience a certain amount of drowsiness—a lazy contented feel, with a strong disinclination to do anything.

Thinking there might be individual differ-

ences of susceptibility to the action of nitro-glycerine, I have laid my friends and others under
contribution, and have induced as many as possible to give it a trial. I have notes of thirty-five
people to whom I have administered it—twelve
males and twenty-three females; their ages varying from twelve to fifty-eight. I find they suffered
from much the same symptoms as I did, although
it affects some people much more than others. Of
the number above quoted, only nine took minim
doses without experiencing decided symptoms.
Women and those below par are much more susceptible to its action than are the strong and robust. A delicate young lady, to whom, adopting
Mr. Field's suggestion, I administered it in drop
doses for the relief of neuralgia, experienced
very decided effects from it, each dose producing
a violent headache lasting from half an hour to
three hours. A married woman, aged thirty-five,
took one minim with very little inconvenience,
but was powerfully affected by two. She was obliged to sit down after each dose, and was positively afraid to move. It made her hot, and caused
such a beating in her head that she had to support
it with her hands. She experienced a heavy weight
on the top of the head, and also a sharp darting
pain across the forehead, which for a moment or
two was very painful to bear. A friend, who for
some days took four drops every three or four
hours, informs me that at times it affected his
head "most strangely." The pulsation was very
distressing, and often lasted an hour or more,
being intensified by moving. It has relieved him
of an old-standing facial neuralgia, and he is en-
thusiastic in its praise. A young woman, aged
twenty-nine, complained that after every dose of

the medicine—one minim—"it seemed as if the top of her head were being lifted off," and this continued sometimes for five minutes, and sometimes longer. The medicine made her bewildered, and she felt sick. A patient with a faint apex systolic murmur was ordered one minim in half an ounce of water four times a day. He took two doses, but it caused "such a beating, thumping, hot pain" in his head that he was unable to continue it. A young man who was given nitro-glycerine in mistake for phosphorus said it made his temples throb, and he could see his pulse beat so distinctly that he was frightened. It caused a burning and flushing in his face, and "took every bit of strength away." This would last for twenty minutes or half an hour after each dose. There was no headache. That alarming symptoms may be produced by large doses, is shown by the following case. A woman, aged fifty-one, was ordered drop-doses of the one per cent solution every four hours. This was taken well, and at the expiration of a week the dose was doubled. No complaint being made, it was then increased to four minims, and after a time to six. The patient said "the medicine agreed with her," and even leading questions failed to elicit any complaint of headache or the like. After the medicine had been taken continuously for five weeks the dose was increased to ten minims. The patient then stated that the medicine no longer agreed with her; it made her sick after every dose and took her appetite away. She always vomited about five minutes after taking the medicine, the vomiting being immediately followed by headache. The medicine made her "go off in a faint" after each dose. She had three "fainting fits" in one day, and could not venture to take another dose. She became quite insensible, and once remained so for ten minutes. Each fainting-fit was "followed by cold shivers," which "shook her violently all over." Her husband and friends were greatly alarmed, but she thought on the whole it had done her good. She had never noticed that the medicine produced drowsiness. In another case a three-minim dose taken on an empty stomach caused a feeling of faintness; "everything goes dark," the patient said, "just as if I were going to faint." The patient could take the same dose after meals without the production of any unpleasant symptom. Drowsiness is not an uncommon result of taking nitro-glycerine. A woman who was given drop-doses four times a day said that she usually went fast asleep immediately after each dose, sleeping from three to four hours. In my own case, the desire for sleep was almost irresistible, although the sleep seldom lasted more than an hour. In exceptional cases none of the ordinary symptoms are exhibited. A man with epispadias —to be presently mentioned—took twenty-five minims of the one per cent solution without any inconvenience.

From a consideration of the physiological action of the drug, and more especially from the similarity existing between its general action and that of nitrite of amyl, I concluded that it would probably prove of service in the treatment of angina pectoris, and I am happy to say that this anticipation has been realised.

As a preliminary step I was anxious to obtain a comparative series of sphygmographic tracings, and for these I am indebted to the kindness and courtesy of Dr. Fancourt Barnes, whose extensive practical acquaintance with the sphygmograph is a guarantee of their accuracy. During the last three months Dr. Barnes has taken over 150 tracings of my pulse, some showing the influence of nitro-glycerine, in others of nitrite of amyl. It would be tedious to describe the observations in detail, more especially as the tracings speak for themselves, and we consequently give only a summary of our results. Judged by the sphygmographic tracings, the effects of nitrite of amyl and of nitro-glycerine on the pulse are similar. Both drugs produce a marked state of dicrotism, and both accelerate the rapidity of the heart's action. They differ, however, in the time they respectively take to produce these effects. The full action of the nitro-glycerine is not observed in the sphygmographic tracings until six or seven minutes after the dose has been taken. In the case of nitrite of amyl the effect is obtained in from fifteen to twenty seconds after an inhalation or a dose has been taken on sugar. The influence of the nitrite of amyl is extremely transitory, a tracing taken a minute and a half after the exhibition of the drug being perfectly normal. In fact, the full effect of the nitrite of amyl on the pulse is not maintained for more than fifteen seconds. The nitro-glycerine produces its effects much more slowly; they last longer, and disappear gradually, the tracing not resuming its normal condition for nearly half an hour. The effect may be maintained for a much longer time by repeating the dose. Nitro-glycerine is more lasting in its power of producing a dicrotic form of pulse-beat, and consequently in cases where the conditions of

Influence of Nitrite of Amyl on the Pulse.

No. 1.—Before inhalation.

No. 3.—Eight minutes after dose.

No. 2.—One minute after inhalation.

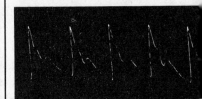

No. 4.—Nine minutes after dose.

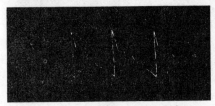

No. 3.—Two minutes after inhalation.

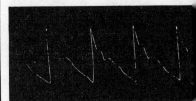

No. 5.—Ten minutes after dose.

Influence of Nitro-Glycerine on the Pulse.

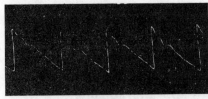

No. 1.—Before dose.

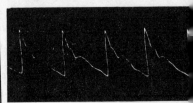

No. 6.—Twenty-two minutes after dose

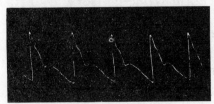

No. 2.—Two minutes after dose.

No. 7.—Twenty-six minutes dose.

relaxation and dicrotism are desired to be maintained for some space of time, its exhibitor is to be preferred to that of nitrite of amyl.

Whilst making some observations with nitro-glycerine on a patient suffering from epispadias, he called attention to the fact that the administration of the drug always caused an increased flow of urine. On examination, fifty-three minutes after the administration of a dose of twelve minims of the one per cent solution, the urine was seen spouting from the extremity of each ureter in a little jet some three or four inches high. Ordinarily the urine dribbles away drop by drop, and never spouts out. The patient was much amazed, and said that in the whole course of his life he had never known it go on in that way. If he took beer or spirits it would increase the flow, but this, to use his own expression, "licked everything." He was made to lie on his face so that all the urine might be collected. In twelve minutes he secreted 6³1/4oz. of urine, the sp. gr. of which was only 1000. He was then given another dose of fifteen minims in a little water, and in the next twelve minutes he secreted 7³1/4oz. Three days later, no nitro-glycerine having been given in the mean time, an observation was made with the view of determining the normal rate of secretion. In half an hour he secreted 3¹1/2oz., the sp. gr. of which was 1005. This, he stated, was more than he usually passed, for he had taken three-quarters of a pint of milk about two hours before, and "it was just running through him."

On another occasion a more systematic observation was made. His urine was collected every quarter of an hour for two hours, patient having had nothing to eat or drink for four hours previously. The quantities passed were as follows:—

1st quarter of an hour,   2¾ drachms.

2nd   ,,   ,,   2¾   ,,

He was then given fifteen minims of the one per cent nitro-glycerine solution in a drachm of water.

3rd quarter of an hour, 12   drachms.

4th   ,,   ,,   16   ,,

5th   ,,   ,,   6¾   ,,

6th   ,,   ,,   8¾   ,,

7th   ,,   ,,   5¾   ,,

8th   ,,   ,,   3   ,,

The times were accurately taken, and in no instance was any of the urine lost. The increased secretion was obviously due to the drug. It is noteworthy that the maximum increase was not till the second quarter. Every specimen was examined as it was passed, and they were all free from sugar and albumen. The quantity was too small to admit of the sp. gr. being taken by the urinometer, except in the case of the fourth quarter, when it was found to be 1003. It should be mentioned that this patient was very insusceptible to the action of the drug, and he experienced none of the ordinary symptoms from this dose.

In another observation on the same patient the results were still more striking. The same method of collecting the urine every quarter of an hour was adopted, and the following figures were obtained:—

			Sp. gr.	Pulse
1st quarter of an hour,	4 dr.	......	–	 64
2nd ” ”	10½ dr.	......	1003	 64

Given twenty minims of one per cent, nitroglycerine in one drachm of water.

			Sp. gr.	Pulse
3rd quarter of an hour,	7 oz.	....	1000	 80
4th ” ”	7½ oz.	....	1000	 76
5th ” ”	1 oz.	....	1002	 72
6th ” ”	7 dr.	....	–	 68
7th ” ”	4½ dr.	....	–	 64

The acidity of the urine varied inversely as the quantity passed. Thus, before the administration of the drug, it was distinctly acid, during the third and fourth quarters it was almost neutral, the acidity then gradually returned, till, in the seventh quarter, it was as marked as it had been at first. No sugar or albumen was detected either before or after the administration of the drug. The figures given under the head of pulse are averages of several observations made during each quarter of an hour. No subjective symptoms of any kind were produced. The experiment was commenced at ten in the morning, and patient had had nothing to eat or drink since breakfast at six. This epispadiac man was curiously insusceptible to the action of the drug as far as subjective symptoms were concerned. I gave him the one per cent nitro-glycerine solution on ten different occasions, in doses of 3, 4, 4, 6, 12, 15, 15, 20, and

25 minims, without causing him a moment's pain or uneasiness. He never complained of headache, or beating or throbbing in any way, and yet the influence, both on the pulse and on the secretion of the urine, was well marked. Even the small doses affected the rate of his pulse. Thus, on one occasion, his pulse was taken every minute for eleven minutes, the average being 68. He was then given a little water in a medicine glass—a practice always followed in these observations— to test the effects of expectoration. The pulse remained constant at 68 during the next five minutes, and 6 minims of the one per cent solution were then given in water. In a minute and a half the pulse had risen to 76, and this increased rate was maintained for the next fifteen minutes, when it sank again to normal. On another occasion his pulse, taken on ten consecutive minutes, was found to be 80. He was then given twenty minims of the one per cent solution in water. Half a minute after the pulse was still 80, in one and a half minutes after it was 96, and in two and a half minutes after it was 100, the average of the eight minutes following the administration of the drug being 96.

Such were the results of the ten series of observations on this man—negative as regards his own sensations. As a final experiment it was decided that he should take a larger dose. At 11.51 A.M., sitting still in the cool laboratory, and having had nothing since an early breakfast, his pulse was 76. At 11.55′ 30″ he took half a drachm of the one per cent solution in a little water. At 11.56, pulse 76; at 11.57, 92; at 11.58, 96, soft and regular. At 12.4 he commenced yawning violently, and said he felt very sleepy. At 12.7 the pulse fell to 68, the yawning ceased, and he became very pale and complained of nausea. He was found to be perspiring freely all over the body, and was so hot that he kicked off his boots. The nausea lasted till 12.10, when the colour had returned to his face, and he said he felt all right again; pulse 76 to 80. There was no headache, and even a sharp run upstairs failed to produce any feeling of pulsation.

During the last nine months I have treated three cases of undoubted angina pectoris with nitro-glycerin, with what success the cases themselves will show.

William A—, aged sixty-four, first came under observation in December, 1877, complaining of intense pain in the chest, excited by the slightest exertion. It was distinctly paroxysmal, patient being perfectly well in the intervals. The first attack was experienced in September, 1876. Patient was at the time in his usual health, and was, in fact, out for a day's pleasure in the country. The pain seized him quite suddenly when walking. It was a most severe attack—as severe a one as ever he experienced in his life. It caused both him and his friends great alarm, and they were most anxious that he should return home at once. He cannot tell at all what brought it on; he had been enjoying himself very quietly; it was not by any means a cold day, and he had not been running, or even walking faster than usual. He remained perfectly well until the following April, when he experienced another similar attack; and since then he has been suffering from them with increasing frequency. From September, 1877, they have been a source of constant anxiety, and it was only by a determined effort that he could continue to follow his occupation.

The attacks usually commence with a feeling of warmth, then of heat, and then of burning heat, in the chest, immediately followed by a heavy pressure, from the midst of which proceeds an acute pain, so that in a moment the whole chest seems as if it were one mass of pain. It is almost impossible, he says, to describe it, for he never felt anything like it before. The pain is first experienced at a small spot on either side of the sternum, corresponding to its junction with the fourth costal cartilages. From the chest the pain flies to the inner side of the arm, at a point midway between the shoulder and the elbow, but never to the fingers. It is not more severe on one side than the other. During the seizure the patient suffers most acutely, and feels convinced that some day he will die in an attack. He usually experiences some shortness of breath at the time, but there is no feeling of constriction about the chest. He can speak during the seizure, though with some difficulty. The attacks are not accompanied by any sensation of warmth or chilliness, but patient is under the impression that he grows pale at the time. These attacks are induced only by exertion in some form or other, most commonly by walking, and especially by walking fast. Walking up hill is sure to bring on a seizure. Stooping down has a similar effect, and the act of pulling on the boots will excite a paroxysm almost to a certainty. He is almost afraid to stoop down, and when he wants to pick up anything from the floor he goes down on his hands and knees. He has a slight cough, but although it shakes him at times it never brings on the pain. The attacks are not excited by food, but exercise taken after meals is more likely to induce them than when taken on an empty stomach. Patient has noticed that they are far more readily excited immediately after breakfast than at any other period of the day. They are more readily induced, too, after an indigestible meal than at other times, but patient is quite clear that no amount of indigestible food *per se* will bring on an attack. The paroxysms, as a rule, last only three or four minutes, but occasionally from twenty minutes to half an hour. If they come on whilst he is walking they always continue till he stops. Patient finds that stimulants afford no relief. In the intervals between the attacks patient is perfectly well, and he feels that if he could only remain absolutely quiet the whole day long he would be quite free from pain. Practically, as he is obliged to be out and about, he has several attacks, on an average six or eight every day. At the time of coming under observation the seizures were rapidly increasing both in frequency and severity. His family history was fairly good. His father died at the age of eighty-three, and hardly had a day's illness in his life. His mother died of phthisis, but only, patient says, through catching cold, hers not being a consumptive family. He lost two brothers—one at the age of eighteen from consumption, and the other in the tropics, cause unknown. He has two brothers and one sister living, all well. There is no family history of gout, asthma, fits, heart disease, or sudden death. He has four children, one of whom (a boy) is consumptive, and another (a girl) subject to facial neuralgia. Patient is a bailiff by occupation, and is a remarkably intelligent man. He is a cool, clear-headed fellow, but little prone to talk of his sufferings, although they are at times very severe. He has travelled much, and has lived in Egypt, Turkey, Italy, and Greece. For the last thirty years he has been accustomed to lead an active out-door life, seldom walking less than fifteen miles a day, often very fast. He has, he says, done a great deal of hard work in the way of pleasure. He usually smokes about two ounces of birds-eye in the week, and has done so for years. His health has always been remarkably good, and, with the exception of rheumatism ten or twelve years ago, and pleurisy seven years ago, he has never known what it is to be laid up. He has never suffered from gout. On a physical examination it is noticed that there is some fibroid degeneration of the arteries, and there is slight hypertrophy of the left ventricle. There are no signs of valvular disease, and there is nothing to indicate the existence of aneurism. The urine was free from albumen.

There could be no possibility of doubt respecting the diagnosis. It was a typical uncomplicated case of angina pectoris.

Patient was placed for a week on infusion of quassia, in order that he might be observed, and also to eliminate the effects of expectation. It need hardly be said that he derived no benefit from this treatment. He was then ordered dropdoses of the one per cent nitro-glycerin solution in half an ounce of water three times a day. At the expiration of a week he reported that there had been a very great improvement. The attacks had been considerably reduced in frequency, and for two or three days he had had only one attack—in the morning after breakfast. The attacks, when they did occur, were much less severe. He found, too, that a dose of medicine taken during an attack would cut it short. He had tried it several times, and it had always succeeded. It would not act instantly, but still very quickly; so that the attacks were considerably shortened. He was thoroughly convinced that the medicine had done him good, and said he was better than he had been since first he had the attacks. It was found that the nitro-glycerin, even in this small dose, had produced its physiological action. Patient complained that for two or three days he had experienced a strange fulness in his head, with a sense of pulsation. The pulsation was felt chiefly in the temples, but also across the forehead. It caused him no positive inconvenience, and he evidently had no suspicion that it was due to the medicine. The dose was then increased to three minims, and patient found that this gave him more speedy relief. On two days during the week he had no seizure at all—a most unusual circumstance. Patient had adopted the plan of carrying his medicine with him in a phial, and taking a dose if an attack seized him in the street. It never failed to afford relief. The beating had increased considerably in intensity, and was described as being a "kind of a pulse." Patient had discovered the fact that it was produced by the medicine. It came on immediately after each dose, and lasted about a quarter of an hour. It was now experienced chiefly across the forehead. Patient continued steadily to improve, and the dose was gradually and cautiously increased. With the increase in dose the pulsation became more severe, lasting from twenty minutes to half an hour. When twelve minims were given every three hours it became a positive inconvenience.

On January 14th the dose of the nitro-glycerin solution was increased to fifteen minims every three hours. A few days later he had a "kind of a fit" immediately after having his medicine. The pulsation came on as usual, but was quickly followed by headache and pain at the back of the neck. His speech "began to go off," and he felt that he would have lost his senses had they not given him tea and brandy.

Patient took the fifteen-minim dose every three hours from the 14th to the 28th of January, but on the latter date had two "bad shocks." He took a dose of medicine in the morning as usual, and felt the customary pulsation, which passed off after about half an hour. An hour and a half later he experienced a sensation as if he would lose his senses. He did not fall, but had to catch hold of something to prevent himself from so doing. It did not last more than half a minute, and there was no pulsation with it. The other seizure occurred later in the day, and was of the same nature. Patient attributed these attacks to the medicine, and was in no way alarmed by them. He thought it advisable, however, to reduce the dose by a third, and henceforth had no return of the fits. At this time his anginal attacks were so thoroughly kept in check by the nitro-glycerin that they gave him comparatively little inconvenience. He always carried his bottle of medicine with him, and immediately on experiencing the slightest threatening of an attack he took a sip. Relief was certain, for even when it did not at once cut short the attack it eased the pain so considerably that he was able to go on walking. For two months longer he continued the ten-minim dose, sometimes taking a little more, and sometimes a little less. He preferred taking it occasionally, as he thought it might be necessary to take it regularly. For the last eight months he has taken nothing but cod-liver oil, and sometimes tonics, and has not had a single attack. He attends once or twice a month, but is perfectly well. He can walk and get about as well as ever he could.

The second case was that of Mrs. H. S—, aged fifty-three, who first came under observation in January, 1878. She is a married woman and the mother of eight children. She complained of a "strange sensation" in her chest, over her heart, coming on in fits several times a day. It was not a pain, she said, at least not an ordinary pain; it was something more than that—it was "just as if the life were going out of her." The attacks would last only two or three minutes at a time, but she seemed as if she could not get her breath, and they frightened her. She could just say "Oh dear!" or something like that, but nothing more. She would usually put her hand over her heart and press hard, and that seemed to relieve her. She feels quite cold during an attack, and her friends tell her she gets pale in the face. The sensation is referred to a spot corresponding in situation to the point of maximum intensity of the heart's beat. It always keeps in the same place, and never flies to the shoulders or runs down the arms. In the intervals of the seizures she is perfectly well. There is no flatulence, nausea, vomiting, numbness in the arms, or vertigo, and the attacks are not followed by any discharge of urine. Patient never has an attack when quiet. The slightest exertion will bring one on; going upstairs will always do so, and even if she goes up very slowly she is sure to get an attack. She does not often get them on level ground. She can always tell, she says, when the ground is rising; she knows directly. Shaking up a bed will bring on the pain at once. She dare not do it now, and that is a great bother to her. Any little exertion is enough, as, for example, putting on her jacket or reaching up to the clothes-line. Stooping down to lift anything brings them on, but not simply stooping down, as in pulling on her boots. Leaning back is certain to bring them on; the least excitement will do so—in fact, anything that worries or upsets her. They are not in any way influenced by food. Cold feet will not bring them on, nor will a hot room. These attacks commenced at the beginning of last summer (1877), but were not so bad as they are now. They worried her a good deal, lasted on and off for two or three months, and then went away. She cannot tell at all what brought them on. They returned on the following November, and have been getting worse ever since. Now she usually has seven or eight attacks a day, but the number depends very much on what she has to do. For some time past they have been gradually increasing in frequency, and are now far more readily excited than formerly. Her general health is fairly good. She has had a bad cough every winter for the last eighteen years. What with the cough and the children, she has never been very strong. She has never suffered from gout or anything like it. Patient's father died of gout and bronchitis. He had suffered from gout since he was twenty-one, and had large chalk stones. He was addicted to drink all his life more or less. His father and brother died of asthma.

Patient's mother died in confinement, and she has no brothers or sisters. She lost one of her children from bronchitis and another from consumption. None of them ever had fits or St. Vitus's dance. On a physical examination, marked arterial degeneration is noticed. There is slight emphysema. There are no signs of aneurism and none of valvular mischief. Urine normal.

Here, again, little doubt was entertained respecting the diagnosis. It was not a typical case of angina pectoris perhaps, but it assimilated more closely to that type of disease than to any other. There could be no doubt about the reality of the patient's sufferings.

After a preliminary course of camphor-water, the patient commenced taking the nitro-glycerin on Feb. 4th. She was ordered one drop of the one percent solution in half an ounce of water every four hours. In three days she reported that the pains had occurred less frequently; that they did not last so long. The pains were much shorter, and "there was a good bit of difference." She complained that the medicine had given her "such a strange sensation." It gave her "a kind of pain inside her head," and brought on a throbbing across her forehead just where the hair begins. After each dose she felt powerless for about ten minutes, and had to sit down, feeling that she could not do anything. The dose was then increased to four minims every four hours, and this gave very marked relief to the anginal symptoms. The pains, she said, were very much better, and a dose of the medicine would always cut them short, almost at once; they were less frequent, less severe, and did not last so long. She was no longer afraid to hurry about the house, and was able to perform many little household duties that had been long neglected. She spoke very positively as to the good the medicine was doing her, but at the same time complained that it affected her most powerfully. The throbbing in her head after the dose was very strong, and lasted nearly twenty minutes; it was accompanied by a darting pain, and she felt cold all over; she had to sit down, and could do nothing as long as it lasted.

The patient continued to improve, and on Feb. 21st she said she had taken a long walk the day before, not only without difficulty, but with pleasure. Under ordinary circumstances the exertion would have brought on an attack, and she would probably have had to return home. The attacks are now experienced only once or twice a day, in spite of her getting about much more; and they are very much slighter than formerly, not lasting half the time. She does not take much notice of them now, and no longer has to stop and put her hand over her heart. Some days she is entirely free from them.

Curiously enough, although the dose of the nitro-glycerine had been gradually increased to ten minims every four hours, the patient complained less of the throbbing in the head. During the following week the dose was increased, first to fifteen and then to twenty minims every four hours. The effect of the larger dose was very marked. She said the medicine made her "feel very bad;" she was afraid of it, for she felt it to her very fingers' ends. She throbbed all over—fingers, toes, and all. It affected her powerfully, and she had to sit down on the bed for nearly three-quarters of an hour after each dose. It caused noises in her ears just like the rushing of water, and made her feel cold all over. Sometimes it produced curious fits of gasping; she went on yawning and yawning, and seemed as if she would never stop. It never made her feel faint, and when it was over she felt quite well again.

The dose of the medicine was now gradually diminished, and on March 7th it was abandoned in favour of general tonics. The patient is still under observation, and, although she has slight attacks occasionally, they give her very little trouble. For the last eight months she has not had a single bad attack of pain.

R. A—, aged sixty-one, a painter's labourer, was first seen on April 11th, 1878. Complains of a pain in the chest, which comes on when he walks. The pain is referred to the mid-sternal region, and is said to cover an area about the size of a teacup. It is a dull, heavy, tight pain. It begins in the chest, and then passes through to between the shoulders. During severe attacks it sometimes runs down the left arm as far as the elbow; it never extends to the lower extremities. It is excited by exertion, and chiefly by walking. It comes on suddenly, and he is obliged to stop and wait till it goes off. He may have to stop for a minute or two, or even longer. It often returns when he starts again. When walking it may come on several times in the course of half an hour, until at last it brings him to a full stop. If he walks fast it will bring it on, and so will going up hill. His ordinary work does not excite it, nor does stooping. He gets it chiefly morning and night, going to and returning from work. Has not noticed that it is more readily induced after meals, and does not think that food influences it in any way. When pain comes on he gets pale, so his friends tell him.

Does not feel anxious, and the attacks do not frighten him at all. They are not accompanied by palpitation, but during the attack he feels "very full," "as if he must burst," or "as if his chest wanted moving." Patient has "knocked about a bit in his time," but has been "fairly steady." First he was on a farm, then in the police, then a wheelwright, and now he is a painter's labourer. When in the police he was advised to resign on account of weakness of his chest, but does not think his chest was really affected, for he had no cough, and has always felt well and strong. Is subject to gout, and had his first attack about three years ago. No history of syphilis. Has been a great smoker for the last forty years; used to smoke an ounce or more nearly every night, especially when on night duty, and it was always shag tobacco, and the strongest he could get. He experienced his first attack twelve years ago, when working on the Thames Embankment. It was the same kind of pain as he has now, but it went off in a week or two. A year later he had a return of it, which lasted for a few weeks. Eight years ago a fire broke out, and he ran a mile and a half to fetch the engines. This brought on the attacks again, and he has had them more or less ever since. He has been getting worse during the last year, and especially during the last few months. On a physical examination, it was found that the pulse was irregular both in force and rhythm. There was some arterial degeneration, and a slight arcus senilis was noticed. No organic disease of the heart or lungs could be detected, and there were no signs of aneurism. Patient had a peculiarly anxious look, which was very noticeable. No albumen in the urine.

After a short course of camphor-water, patient
was ordered a drop of the one per cent solution of
nitro-glycerine in half an ounce of water, to be
taken every four hours. Four days later the patient reported that there had been a great improvement. The attacks were much less frequent,
and that morning he had walked to his work
without having a single seizure—a thing he had
not done before for he could not say how long.
The attacks at night, going home, were just as
frequent, and he did not think they were less
severe when they did come on. He had never
taken a dose of the medicine when the attack was
on him, so he could not say if it would cut it short.
After each dose of the medicine he gets a pain at
the back of the head, which comes on in about ten
minutes and lasts half an hour. Says it is almost
the same kind of pain as he has in his chest—"a
heavy, dull pain"; no beating or throbbing; no
pain across the forehead or at the top of the head.
Sometimes gets a "choky sensation in the throat"
after the medicine. A few days later patient called
again, and stated that he was steadily improving.
At this visit he was given a single dose of two
drops of the one per cent solution on a piece of
sugar. It produced slight flushing of the face and
a marked increase in the fulness of the arteries.
The pulse, which had previously been 98, rapidly
rose to 112. The flushing was in a few minutes
followed by intense pallor, and patient complained of feeling faint. He had to be supported
to the sofa, his pulse was found to be very feeble,
and it was a quarter of an hour or more before he
was sufficiently recovered to stand alone. The
patient was directed to continue the one-drop
dose every four hours, and to take an extra dose

when he felt the pain coming on. A week later he said he thought he was nearly well. For four days he had not had a single attack, although he had had a great deal of walking to do. When he felt any indication of the onset of the pain, he took a sip of his medicine, and it was all gone in a moment. He could walk to his work without the slightest difficulty, and even coming home at night gave him no trouble. The other day he walked the best part of a mile in a shower of rain quite briskly, and was none the worse for it. After each dose he experiences a pain at the back of the head and also over the forehead. A week later the dose was increased to two minims every four hours, and this was taken without difficulty. The medicine, he said, did not upset him at all. It had done him a deal of good, and he did not know what he should do without it. The dose was gradually and cautiously increased to eight minims every four hours. This was taken without difficulty, patient remarking that it did not upset him as it used to do. He was quite free from the attacks as long as he continued taking the medicine, but they returned immediately if he discontinued it. He still attends at long intervals to report himself, but is practically well.

In the following case, of which an abstract of the notes is given, the administration of nitro-glycerin was attended with success.

L. B—, soap-maker, aged forty-two. Complains of pain in the chest on the left side, constant, but increased by movement, very severe at times, and occasionally so acute as to make him cry out; seems as if it would take his breath away; sometimes occurs between the shoulders as well, and not unfrequently runs down the left arm as far as the elbow. If walking, and the pain comes on, he has to stop, but only for a few seconds, and then goes on again. The pain is increased by stooping down, as in putting on his boots. Any movement, even turning in bed, will bring on the acute pain; but still he is never entirely free from it. He has it more or less all day, and acutely on moving. He has the very greatest difficulty in doing his work. Has been abstemious all his life; a smoker, but not consuming more than half an ounce of tobacco a week. Has had gout thirty times or more during the last twelve years. Has had winter cough for about the same time. Never had these pains until this year. Has been gradually losing flesh for some months past. Physical signs those of emphysema; heart normal; no albumen in the urine. The patient was ordered a gentian-and-soda mixture, and this he took for a fortnight without the slightest benefit. The medicine, he said, did him more harm than good. The local application of belladonna failed to afford relief. He was then given drop doses of the one per cent nitro-glycerine solution in half an ounce of water four times a day. A week later he reported that he had felt relief on the first day, and had steadily improved ever since. He could stoop down without getting the old attacks, and could walk about almost as well as ever. He had not the slightest difficulty in taking the medicine. He remained under observation for some time longer, but there was no return of the pain.

In conclusion, I have to thank Dr. Ringer for his kindness in having frequently examined these patients, and also for many valuable suggestions.

REPORT ON THE USE AND EFFECT OF APPLICATIONS OF NITRATE OF SILVER TO THE THROAT

BY HORACE GREEN, M.D.

Reprinted from Transactions of the American Association of Physicians 9: 493-530, 1856

Many years ago the celebrated Abernethy published to the world his treatise "On the Constitutional Origin of Local Diseases." His views have been pronounced enlightened and philosophical; and perhaps justly so. Certainly they were eminently suggestive, for they contributed, more than those of any other writer of that period, to awaken among both surgeons and physicians a spirit of enlightened inquiry with regard to primary diseased action.

But the great work needed now more than any other, by both branches of the profession, and which might be termed, perhaps, the converse of that of Mr. Abernethy, is one which would embrace a full, enlightened, and philosophical history of the *Local Origin of Constitutional Diseases.* Until this neglected portion of the history of Medicine shall have been written by some second Abernethy, thoroughly enlightened and imbued with the vast importance of his subject, the value of topical medication, its effects and utility, cannot be fully appreciated by the profession.

A brief history, only, of the therapeutic effects of a single agent locally employed in the treatment of disease, is doubtless the one expected by those from whom the appointment to report on this subject emanated; and yet the diseases in which topical medication has been already successfuly employed, embrace a wide range, and include many of the most important affections which the physician is called upon to treat. Besides all that has been written in this country on the topical employment of nitrate of silver, several works of some magnitude, besides many monographs, have been published in Europe within a few years, which are devoted wholly or in part, to the history of the effects of this therapeutic agent in the treatment of disease. In reporting, therefore, on this subject, I shall refer primarily and mainly to the views and conclusions of others—to those which appear to be based on carefully recorded observations—believing that the value of my own views and opinions will be enhanced when these are sustained by the experience and the corroborative testimony of distinguished observers of my own and of other countries.

Among the works which have been published on topical treatment, or in which the use of nitrate of silver as a local therapeutic agent is discussed, are the following: "*Dysphonia Clericorum, or Clergyman's Sore Throat, its Pathology and Treatment.* By James Mackness, M.D., member of the College of Physicians, London, &c., published in London, 1848." "*A Treatise on Diseases of the Larynx and Trachea, and their Treatment by the Local Application of Caustics.* By John Hastings, M.D.,

Licentiate of the Royal College of Physicians, London, &c., 1850."

A work on the Medication of the Larynx and Trachea, by S. Scott Allison, M. D., Member of the Royal College of Physicians, London, was published in 1853. And in the same year, Prof. Bennett, of Edinburgh, published his work on Tuberculosis and on the Local Medication of Pharyngeal and Laryngeal Diseases.

But the most comprehensive and valuable publication on this subject, is the recent work of Dr. Watson, of Glasgow, Professor of the Institutes of Medicine in the Andersonian University, in which he declares his object has been to explain the rationale, and to recommend the practice of topical medication to the larynx, not only in those diseases which affect that organ simply and alone, but also in others during the progress of which it is secondarily involved in morbid action.[1]

There are two other foreign works, having reference to diseases of the air-passages and their topical treatment, of which I might speak, both of which were published in London in 1851. The one by a member of the Royal College of Surgeons of England, the other by a Fellow of the Medical Society of London, &c. But as these volumes contain nothing on this subject, not recorded in my own work on *Diseases of the Air-passages*, published in 1846, I shall only allude to them in order to say, that however just the English may have been in accusing American writers of "pirating" and of borrowing largely from English authors, they are themselves not altogether immaculate in this respect. One of these authors has taken copiously from the above work, without the ordinary acknowledgment; whilst the other has made up a good-looking volume of nearly two hundred pages, on *Diseases of the Mucous Membrane of the Throat and their Treatment by Topical Medication*, a large proportion of which in its chapters on pathology, etiology, and treatment, is abstracted from my work; page after page of matter having been copied literally, without any intimation whatever as to its true paternity, and that too without those revisions and improvements which might have been made advantageously, with almost every sentence purloined.

Although many brief articles on the treatment of several of the diseases of the air-passages by means of cauterization, have from time to time appeared in our Medical Journals, yet no work, not even a monograph, especially devoted to this subject, has ever been published by any one among my own countrymen.

Among the diseases, in the treatment of which the preceding authors have recommended the employment of applications of nitrate of silver, are the following: Follicular disease of the pharyngo-laryngeal mucous membrane, acute and chronic laryngitis, croup, edema of the glottis, aphonia, hooping-cough, spasmodic asthma, chronic bronchitis, laryngismus, and tuberculosis, especially when the latter affection is consequent on or complicated with laryngeal disease.

Now, the question very appropriately presents itself, on what principle in national or scientific medicine, is that practice founded by which several diseases, diverse in their indications, can be successfully treated by the employment of a single topical remedy?

Dr. Watson, in his recent valuable work, to which I have alluded, in considering the *modus*

operandi of this local stimulant, in the treatment
of inflammations of the mucous membrane, of-
fers an interesting rationale of that treatment,
showing its applicability to many diseases, which
at first sight are essentially different; "as different, for example, as hooping-cough and laryngitis, or as either of these and aphonia."

All practitioners who have used this local
remedy to any extent, have found it highly
important to vary the strength of the solution in
different cases, and also according to the condition of the diseased membrane. When a solution
of nitrate of silver of moderate strength is applied
to the mucous membrane, it acts chemically on
the mucus with which it comes in contact, and
throws down a copious white deposit that coats
the membrane beneath.

"In erosion and ulceration of the mucous membrane," says Dr. Watson, "the deposit of the white
substance before alluded to, from the caustic solution, is thickened by coagulation of the albumen
of the *liquor sanguinis*, which transudes from the
exposed vessels, and thus protection is afforded
to the delicate and inflamed parts beneath."[1] The
therapeutic effect which follows the stimulation
produced in the vessels of the parts, by the application of the argentine solution, he explains by a
reference to the action of this remedy, on the
different degrees and stages of that inflammatory process, which is artificially produced in the
web of a frog's foot, stretched out under a micro-
scope.

When, for example, he says, "a red-hot needle
is passed through the web, the following are the
phenomena observed: A spot in the centre of the
inflamed part is sphacelated, destroyed by the

passage of the needle through it; a circle around
the spot is usually found in a state of complete
congestion, the vessels being dilated and the cor-
puscles almost perfectly stationary within them,
while in the part beyond this circle, the vessels are
not so much dilated, and the stasis of their contents is not so complete. The stream is seen
passing slowly away into the collateral circulation
of the unaffected parts of the web."

"Now these two circles represent two degrees
of inflammation, which it is important to distin-
guish wherever they occur and perhaps especially
when the seat of morbid action is the mucous
membrane of the larynx or trachea. That part of
the web of the frog's foot in which the stasis was
complete, represents the most intense, or sthenic
degree; the other, in which the stasis was not so
complete, represents what is usually called the
subacute, and perhaps chronic varieties. And the
effects of the solution of caustic on each of these
parts, is markedly and importantly different. In
the part which is most intensely inflamed, the
solution in the direct ratio of its strength increases
the stasis of the blood within the vessels. The
latter seem to be unable to dilate further, and are,
therefore, little changed, but the nitrate of silver
acts through the coats upon the blood which they
contain by causing its partial coagulation, and
likewise by withdrawing water from the serum
for the crystals of the nitrate which begin partially
to form if the solution is strong. In that part of the
web, on the other hand, which had been less
intensely inflamed, the stimulant solution causes
a renewed and increased dilatation of the bloodvessels, and the retarded current moves on in
them more freely than before; a cure being thus

speedily effected if the exciting cause of the inflammation had ceased to act."[1]

From these experiments Dr. Watson believes we are warranted in concluding that the purely stimulant action of this remedy is beneficial, in all varieties of the inflammatory process, except the most intense; and that a strong solution not only stimulates the vessels, but tends, as in the different varieties of oedema, to remove the watery part of their contents, on the laws of *exosmose* and *endosmose*.

Prof. Bennett, of Edinburgh, on the other hand, declares in his recent work on *Pulmonary Tuberculosis*, that "the action of the nitrate of silver solution is not that of a stimulant, but rather that of a calmative or sedative. It acts chemically on the mucous, pus, or other albuminous fluids it comes in contact with, throws down a copious white precipitate, in the form of a molecular membrane, which defends, for a time, the tender mucous surface, or irritable ulcer, and leaves the passage free for acts of respiration. Hence the feeling of relief almost always occasioned; that diminution of irritation in the parts, which is so favorable to cure, and why it is that strong solutions of the salt are much more efficacious than weak ones."[2]

Dr. Scott Alison, in his work on the *Medication of the Larynx and Trachea*, expresses the opinion that the nitrate of silver, when applied to an acutely inflamed organ, is an irritant, and may aggravate the morbid condition. "To a part affected with chronic inflammation," he says, "it is a tonic and a stimulant, and therefore is likely to be beneficial. To a tissue, the subject of irritation, it is a sedative. Applied to a membrane, which for some time has been the seat of excessive and unhealthy secretion, it abates and corrects it."[3]

These are the opinions of a few of the distinguished members of the profession—men who have had the largest experience in the use of the remedy—of the therapeutic action of the nitrate of silver solution, in the treatment of diseases of the lining membrane of the air-tubes.

I shall now proceed, in as brief a manner as possible, to specify some of the most important of the local and general diseases which have been enumerated, in the treatment of which, the Use and Effect of Nitrate of Silver have been observed and recorded.

1st. *The Effect of Nitrate of Silver in the Treatment of Follicular Pharyngo-laryngeal Disease.*

In advocating the employment of topical me dication, in the treatment of diseases of the air-passages, in the work to which I have alluded, I state that, "in the simple and uncomplicated form of follicular pharyngo-laryngeal disease, however severe the local affection may have been, this remedy alone, namely, the crystals of nitrate of silver topically applied, has proved in my hands a specific in a large number of cases."[1]

This opinion of the efficacy of the remedy in this disease, has been fully sustained by subsequent experience, in the practice of many distinguished physicians in this and in other countries. It is well known that Prof. Bennett, of the University of Edinburgh, has adopted extensively topical medication in the treatment of laryngeal and kindred diseases, in the Royal Infirmary, and in his private practice.

In his treatise on *Pulmonary Tuberculosis and*

Laryngeal Affections, much valuable information
on this subject, and many interesting cases, successfully treated by the applications of nitrate of
silver, are given. I shall take the liberty of noting
the following

CASE.—"I was requested by an assurance office, in July, 1850, to examine the chest of Mr.
M—, a merchant, aged about 30, who said he
labored under no kind of complaint, with the
exception of occasional sore throat, and expectoration of mucus tinged with blood. He was tolerably stout, took long walks without uneasiness,
and suffered from no difficulty of respiration or
from cough. Repeated examination of his chest
failed to elicit any physical sign indicative of pulmonary disease. I therefore certified that his
lungs were healthy. In October, 1851, this gentleman called upon me again for advice, under the
following circumstances. The soreness of the
throat had latterly increased, and considerable
cough was induced, after which he spat up
mouthfuls of purulent matter, frequently tinged
of a red color. He brought me some of this
sputum to examine, which consisted of mixed
blood and pus, of a dirty brick-red color. Examination of his chest again convinced me that the
lungs were unaffected; but in the interval I had
paid attention to the writings and practice of Dr.
Horace Green, of New York; and I now examined his throat, when the cause of his symptoms was at once apparent. The fauces and upper
part of the pharynx were studded over with
nodular swellings, varying in size from a pin head
to that of a pea. Many of them were bright red,
and fungoid in character, probably the origin of
the extravasated blood, whilst considerable

patches of purulent matter adhered to several parts of the mucous membrane. I applied a sponge, saturated with a strong solution of the nitrate of silver, to the affected parts. In three days he returned, having been much relieved, when the application was repeated. I have not seen him since.

"These two cases (a second case being recorded by Dr. B., not quoted) convinced me that certain symptoms which have hitherto been considered as indicative of phthisis, might have their origin entirely in the fauces, pharynx, and upper part of the larynx. The cough, so occasioned, with the purulent expectoration, often tinged with blood, frequently so resembles that occasioned by phthisis, as not only to induce alarm in the minds of the patients, but frequently to mislead the medical practitioner. I have now met with many such cases, which have been mistaken for phthisis, and which have been treated for that disease without any effect, until local remedies were applied, when they, for the most part, disappeared or became much better."[1]

Dr. Bennett enumerates other cases of follicular disease, where all the symptoms of phthisis pulmonalis were present, including emaciation, profuse sweating, cough, expectoration of pus mingled with blood, bad appetite, hectic; and, in consequence, cod-liver oil, cough mixtures, acid drops, wine and good diet were administered, and all without effect; "but which in many instances were cured by the topical applications."

2d. *The Effect of Nitrate of Silver in the Treatment of Acute and Chronic Laryngitis.*

Dr. Hastings, in his excellent *Treatise on Dis-*

eases of the Larynx and Trachea, expresses great confidence in the use of the Nitrate of Silver, as a local remedy in the treatment of these affections; and he also details many cases of much interest, in which topical medication proved effectual in arresting the disease, after other measures had failed. Under the head of "Follicular Laryngitis," Dr. Hastings alludes to a pathological condition of the larynx and trachea, which, as an independent affection, is very generally overlooked by the profession, or, is considered the sequel—not, as it often is, the antecedent of tuberculosis. "I am satisfied," says Dr. Hastings, "that cases presenting the morbid appearances in the pharynx and arch of the fauces just described, form but a small proportion of those denominated follicular laryngitis."[1] * * * *

"I have repeatedly met with cases in which the disease was confined to those parts, and the back of the velum, where nothing more was required than to carry the solution of the nitrate of silver behind the uvula into the posterior nares, and over the pharynx and fauces, in order to remove a very troublesome cough; whilst in others, and by far the greater number, the disease exists in the larynx and trachea, the fauces and pharynx at the same time presenting a healthy appearance.

"Such cases are, generally, most puzzling to the practitioner. The patient is troubled with cough, the expectoration is muco-purulent, occasionally streaked with blood, to a considerable amount; pains are felt in the chest below the clavicles, he wastes a little, or he may not lose flesh. His chest is examined again and again, but no disease can be discovered; his mouth and throat are inspected without anything being found there to account for the symptoms; at length the disease is regarded as an obscure case of phthisis; he gets treated with sedatives, expectorants, and cod-liver oil, until the ensuing winter, when all his former symptoms return in an aggravated degree, whilst as the warm season comes on, they improve."

"Much pain and suffering might be spared in these cases, were a stethoscopic examination of the windpipe resorted to, which in most cases would point out the nature, situation, and extent of the disease; and the practitioner would have that satisfaction in treating the case, which an imperfect knowledge, or an entire ignorance of it can never give."[2]

Such cases are reported by Dr. Hastings as having been successfully treated by the repeated application of the sponge, saturated with a solution of the nitrate of silver, and which was "carried down the windpipe," he says, "as low as the bifurcation of the bronchi."[1]

In speaking of the practicability of this operation, and of the benefit to be derived from topical medication in disease of the larynx, Prof. Bennett declares, that if the probang be properly prepared, and the operation well performed, the sponge saturated with the solution of nitrate of silver may be rapidly thrust through the rima into the larynx and frequently into the trachea. "I am persuaded," he continues, "that on many occasions, I have passed it pretty deep into the trachea, not only from the length of the probang which has disappeared, but also from the sensations of the patient.[2] * * * In this first part of the operation, the rima glottidis is, as it were, taken by surprise, and the sponge enters, if the right direction be given to it, without difficulty; the rima glottidis immediately contracts by reflex action, so that on withdrawing the instrument you feel the contraction."

"This also squeezes out the solution, which is diffused over the laryngeal and tracheal mucous membrane. Now if the sponge be a fine one, it will be found capable of holding about a half a drachm of fluid, the effect of which upon the secretions and mucous surfaces, almost always produces temporary relief to the symptoms, and strengthens the tone of the voice; results at once apparent after the momentary spasm has abated."

In the treatment of both varieties of chronic laryngitis, the idiopathic and the tubercular, topical applications of the nitrate of silver solution have proved, in the hands of many practitioners, a most efficient and valuable remedy.

Dr. Cotton, one of the physicians of Brompton Hospital, in the work to which I have alluded, in speaking of topical medication in chronic laryngitis and laryngeal phthisis, candidly admits his previous unbelief in, and changed views with regard to the practicability or propriety of topical medication to the mucous membrane of the respiratory passages. The admission is honorable to himself, and worthy of imitation. "I should here remark," he observes, "that my own views upon this subject differ from those I formerly held and have even expressed; and that I owe this change to the kindness of Dr. Horace Green, of New York, the justly celebrated advocate of this treatment, who, during a recent visit to our metropolis, convinced myself and others, not only of the possibility, but of the safety and usefulness of the practice.

"I had long been in the habit of using a solution of nitrate of silver to the pharynx and upper surface of the epiglottis, by means of a soft brush, in all the early cases, both of pharyngeal and laryngeal complication; and had frequently witnessed its good effects, not only upon the part to which it was immediately applied, but upon the laryngeal structures also, attributing it in the latter case to an action excited in the upper respiratory passages from continuity. But I had never ventured to apply anything directly to the larynx itself; not from misgivings as to its effects, but from apprehensions of its danger. For some months past, however, I have done so, extensively in cases of chronic laryngitis, whether idiopathic or tubercular, and very frequently with marked success.

"At the commencement of the laryngeal symptoms, a solution of the crystals of nitrate of silver, varying in strength from ten grains to half a drachm to the ounce of distilled water, passed by means of the instrument recommended by Dr. Green, into the opening of the larynx, is often productive of great relief. I have known the voice regained, the irritable cough removed, and the tenderness and difficulty of swallowing dissipated entirely by it; indeed, I think we might almost speak of its *curative* effects, so far, at least, as the larynx is concerned, in some very early cases."[1]

"In the treatment of acute laryngitis," says Dr. Hastings, "the topical application of a solution of the nitrate of silver may sometimes be employed with great advantage; indeed, unaided, it will not unfrequently remove the disease, but then the patient must be seen sufficiently early.

"If the inflammation has not penetrated into the trachea, but is confined to the larynx, we may safely and successfully venture to employ this topical application; for although a small spot of intense inflammation may be safely and successfully treated in this way, a large surface is irritated by the same means.

"This treatment would not interfere or prevent the use of any additional remedies, such as calomel, opium, aperients, &c." "But it is in the chronic form of laryngitis," Dr. Hastings continues, "that this treatment is remarkably useful. Many such cases improve rapidly under local treatment applied to the larynx and trachea, which, if neglected for months, or it may be for years, not unfrequently lead to permanent changes."[1]

In this connection Dr. Hastings relates some most interesting cases of chronic laryngitis, attended with hoarseness, cough, emaciation, "expectoration streaked with blood," difficulty of breathing, night-sweats, and most of the ordinary symptoms of phthisis—all of which were promptly and permanently relieved by a solution of nitrate of silver of the ordinary strength applied to the larynx and trachea.[2] With regard to the treatment of *tubercular laryngitis*, Dr. Hastings remarks, "I know of no means so capable of arresting and removing it, as sponging the windpipe with a solution of the nitrate of silver.[3]

In the treatment of the non-exudative variety of chronic laryngitis, Dr. Watson has employed and recommends the application of the nitrate of silver to the inflamed mucous membrane; but he considers that a great amount of discrimination is necessary in the adaptation of the strength of the solution to the severity of the inflammation which may be present; as well as in the preparation for commencing the topical measures. In the severe forms of the affection, he believes that depletion of some kind will at first be necessary to check the violence of the inflammation before the applications of the caustic solution are made to the laryngeal membrane;[4] and with regard to the strength of the remedy employed he maintains, that the more intense the degree of inflammation of the laryngeal lining, the weaker ought to be the solution of the nitrate of silver applied to it.[5]

After the intensity of the primary inflammation has been subdued by appropriate treatment, a stronger solution may be used with advantage. "Its first effect," he continues, "when thus judiciously applied, will be to coagulate the albuminous film upon the surface of the membrane which had been stripped of its epithelium, and to secrete new mucus, and thus the artificial film of coagulated albumen is by and by replaced by a more natural covering, and the surface is lubricated by its appropriate moisture.

"If, then, a renewal of the morbid process could be prevented, a cure would already have been effected, but this is seldom or never the case. The good effects of the topical application wear off in a few hours, and the former abnormal phenomena may even in that time have reappeared in nearly equal severity. The treatment must therefore be continued; the touching of the larynx must be repeated frequently for some days; and indeed, until all the symptoms of laryngitis have completely disappeared."[1]

Many practitioners both in this country and in Europe, differ entirely from Dr. Watson, with regard to the strength of the solution to be employed in the treatment of the different degrees of inflammation of the mucous membrane. The weaker solutions, they believe, those for example of the strength of five, ten, or fifteen grains to the ounce of water, act as a stimulant, or as an irritant when applied to a highly inflamed membrane; while a strong solution, by the chemical changes it effects, will prove a sedative, and thus tend directly to subdue the violence of the inflammatory action.

On this point, as we have seen, Prof. Bennett expresses the decided opinion after much observation and experience in the topical use of the nitrate of silver solution, in the treatment of inflammations of the lining membrane of the larynx and trachea, that strong solutions of the salt, by acting as a calmative or sedative, diminish the irritability of the inflamed parts, and are therefore much more efficacious than weak ones.[2]

Dr. Watson, in his treatise, has devoted many pages to the consideration of chronic laryngitis. "In the treatment of chronic disease of the laryngeal mucous membrane," he remarks, "I place my chief reliance on topical applications to the parts affected, but I do not undervalue or neglect more general measures." The strength of the solution, he adds, "should vary with the requirements of the case, and it should be applied every day, or every second day, according to the patient's feelings."[3]

Dr. Alison, in the work to which I have referred, on the *Medication of the Larynx and
Trachea*, details his experience in the employment of other agents beside nitrate of silver, for
the treatment of local diseases; such as At-
rophine, Daturine, Iodine, &c., but he gives the
preference to the first named remedy, as the one
most efficient. "I had so frequently found," he
remarks, "in the treatment of local disease, and
local complications, that many remedies were far
more efficacious, when applied immediately to
the part affected or to its vicinity, than at a distance, that I was glad to learn that a sponge
loaded with the solution of the nitrate of silver,
and affixed to a probang, could not only without
injury but with manifest advantage be passed
through the glottis and the larynx down into the
trachea."[1]

In acute inflammation of the glottis, Dr. Alison
has hesitated to apply the solution, lest "the
presence of the stimulant on parts suffering from
such attacks," might aggravate the disease; but in
chronic inflammations of the larynx, "and of the
upper portion of the trachea, the solution of the
nitrate of silver, he observes, has in my hands as in
others, been very useful in bringing the disease to
a conclusion; and where that has not been accomplished by reason of its dependence upon incurable disease of the lungs, it has almost invariably
afforded very considerable relief, by rendering
the cough less violent and frequent, and removing much of the tickling and uneasy sensations, at
the upper portion of the larynx." * * * * "In some
cases of disease of the larynx and trachea," he
continues, "in which the symptoms inclined to the
suspicion that ulceration existed, the same local

application of a solution of the nitrate of silver has been very useful."[2]

Abundant testimony from many other sources might be gathered, if necessary, to prove the great advantage to be obtained from the topical use of this remedy, in the treatment of laryngeal and tracheal disease.

3d. *The Effects of the Application of Nitrate of Silver in the Treatment of Membranous Croup.*

As a difference of opinion obtains, to some extent, among the profession, with regard to the propriety of employing topical applications of the nitrate of silver in *exudative laryngitis*, or croup, I shall examine with some care the opinions and observations of those who have had extensive opportunities to test its efficacy in the treatment of this, often, fatal malady.

According to the testimony furnished by Prof. Trousseau, of Paris, M. Bretonneau, the preceptor of Trousseau, was the first to employ topical medication in the treatment of membranous croup. Prof. Trousseau, in a letter which I received from him, and which was published in the January number of the *American Medical Monthly*, thus writes: "As early as 1818, Mr. Bretonneau, in the treatment of croup, carried over the aryteno-epiglottic ligaments, several times a day, a sponge fastened to the extremity of a piece of whalebone and charged either with pure chlorohydric acid, or with a saturated solution of nitrate of silver. He expressed the fluid from the sponge at the entrance of the larynx, and the patient in the convulsive movements of respiration caused a certain quantity of the caustic solution to enter therein."[1]

In 1830, M. Trousseau employed for the first time caustic applications in the treatment of disease of the larynx. "I made use," says M. Trousseau, "precisely of the same process which I have pointed out above, in the treatment of croup, and I endeavored to express the caustic solution into the cavity of the larynx." In this connection Prof. Trousseau asserts, "that never, either before or since the publication of your labors, have I attempted to introduce into the larynx or trachea, a sponge saturated with a caustic solution." * * * "and consequently," he continues, "the direct introduction of the sponge saturated with a caustic solution, into the larynx and into the bronchial tubes, does not belong to me in any respect whatever."[2]

This local agent has also been employed after the manner of Bretonneau, in the treatment of pseudo-membranous croup, by MM. Dupuytren, Guersant, Guiet, Bouchut, Berton, and other French practitioners, but no one of the number made any attempt to pass the sponge probang into the larynx.

M. Bouchut, whose work on *Diseases of Children* was published in 1845, advises the employment of cauterizations, in the treatment of the disease, but he observes and recommends great caution in making the applications to the pharynx, and over the glottis, lest too large a quantity of the fluid *should drop into the larynx, and produce suffocation and death*, or at least render it necessary to practice immediate tracheotomy. The following are M. Bouchut's remarks on this subject: "Si la cauterization de l'arrére—bouche et de la partie supérieure du larynx est avantageuse, elle a aussi ses inconvénients qu'il faut connaître pour tacher de les éviter. La suffocation immediate peut en être la consequence, si l'on a laissé trop long temps ,'éponge sur la glotte, et si une trop grande quantité de liquide a pénétré dans la larynx. Cet accident est fort grave, car il peut déterminer la mort, ou au moins la nécessité de pratiquer aussitôt la trachéotomie."[3]

A late number of the *Archives Générales de Médecine* contains an interesting Memoir, by M. Vauthier, on the history of Croup, as it occurred in an epidemic form, in *L'Hôpital des Enfants Malades de Paris*. In this paper are the details of several well marked cases of membranous croup, which were treated successfully by "emetics and cauterizations;" and although in these instances, the argentine solution was not conveyed into the larynx, but was applied only to the fauces and pharynx, yet the patients recovered perfectly under the treatment.[1] Although the cases thus treated are characterized as having been very severe—"trés intense"—yet, as the treatment was early adopted, it is probable that the exudative process had not extended into the larynx; for, in the same paper is a history given, of five other cases of membranous croup, in which the disease, having reached the larynx, was not arrested by cauterizations. This method was employed, as in the other cases, but no attempt was made to pass the instrument below the epiglottis. Tracheotomy, however, was resorted to in all these five cases, but every patient died. Efficient cauterization of the larynx, we maintain, would have saved three, if not more of these last cases.

Among the English practitioners, of whose works, on topical medication, we have spoken, a few only appear to have employed this remedy in the treatment of true exudative croup. Dr. Watson's experience, in the treatment of the few cases he has reported in his work, has led him to the conclusion, "that the topical treatment is unsuitable during the acute stage of exudative croup."

Having been unsuccessful in the management of a single case of membranous croup,[2] in which he employed the treatment through the acute or inflammatory stage of the disease, Dr. Watson adopts and promulgates the above opinion. In the commencement of the disease, or in that stage of the affection denominated by him "the pre-exudative stage of croup," Dr. Watson highly recommends the application of the solution of nitrate of silver to the throat and larynx. Omitting the applications during the acute stage of the disease, he renews the topical measures, as soon as the inflammatory process has been subdued by appropriate reducing measures. But his views on this subject will be best understood from the following brief extract from his work: "There is a large class of cases, in which the croup commences by a longer or shorter stage of simple, though severe inflammation of the laryngeal membrane. This inflammation differs in nothing from the most intense degree of catarrh, formerly described; but it speedily ends either in exudation upon the surface of the membrane, or in serous effusion beneath it.

"The suddenness of the attack, the anxiety of the patient, the severity of the constitutional fever, and above all, the stethoscopic signs of a dry and tense glottis, never fairly released at any stage of respiration, are the chief diagnostic marks of the danger to be expected in the next stage of the disease. No one who has ever listened attentively

to the peculiarly harsh sounds transmitted
through the stethoscope placed over the thyroid
cartilage of a patient in the critical state we are
now considering, can either forget or mistake the
prolonged and dry, but vibratory sound during
inspiration, immediately followed by the less
noisy, though still grating murmur of obstructed
expiration by which it is characterized. Then the
stifling and painful cough, without expectoration, and the whispering, not hoarse voice, are
equally characteristic.

"In children, or in adults predisposed to the
disease, such a group of symptoms as that just
referred to, may be considered as certainly indicative of the first stage of exudative croup. But no
exudation has yet been poured out, and, according to my experience, the disease may here
be checked by the application of an appropriately
strong solution of the nitrate of silver; and I will
venture to assert it is in the treatment of this pre-
exudative stage of croup, if I may be allowed so to
name it, for sake of brevity, that Dr. Horace
Green has also been successful."

This abortive treatment of croup by topical
applications, is further illustrated by Dr. Watson,
in his relation of the subjoined case: "It is that of a
family of young children," he says, "all of whom
are remarkably subject to croup, and, notwithstanding the utmost care in their management,
some of them have suffered once or twice from
the disease during the winter, for some years
past. In the beginning of the present year, I attended two of them, and, within the last few days,
a third, when attacked by this disagreeable
visitant.

" Whenever a croupy cough is heard in this

family, the throat and larynx are at once touched with the solution of caustic. A warm bath, a few drops of antimonial wine, and, if necessary, a dose of laxative medicine, are next had recourse to, and very little else is generally required. The throat is touched for the two or three succeeding days, by which time the child is usually quite well.

"Only once that I remember did this abortive treatment fail in my hands, and it was in the case of a member of the family here referred to. The weather was at the time very severe, and the subject of the disease, a strong little boy about six years of age. For some reason or other, it was longer than usual, too, before the topical application was made to the larynx, and it failed. Exudation was thrown out, and the boy passed through a critical illness, during the intensity of which I laid aside the topical treatment, and employed leeches, calomel, and antimony. But when, as happily occurred in this case, the exudation had separated in due time, I renewed the stimulant applications to the windpipe, with marked benefit, and the child made a speedy and perfect recovery."

In one other respect Dr. Watson differs from most practitioners in this country, namely, in the strength of the solution which he employs in the treatment of croup. He has found in practice, he says, that a solution "of fifteen or twenty grains to the ounce of water, is abundantly successful in fulfilling the indications of the disease."[2]

Although a prejudice against the local treatment is still entertained by many practitioners, applications of the nitrate of silver in the treatment of membranous croup have been employed, with more or less success, by physicians in

every part of this country. Contributions from
the profession have been made from time to time
to most of our medical journals, during the last
ten years, in which cases successfully treated by
this agent are detailed. I will refer only to the
opinion and observations of one of these writers;
a distinguished permanent member of this Association; it is well known to the reading members
of the profession, that several years ago, Dr.
Ware, of Boston, published his contributions to
the "History and Diagnosis of Croup,"—a work
evincing more scientific research, and containing
more information with regard to the true pathology of membranous croup, than all that had previously been written in America. In these papers,
Dr. Ware refers to thirty-nine cases of what he
denominates membranous croup, which were
noticed in his own, or in the practice of his
friends. Of these cases the state of the fauces was
observed in thirty-three instances, and "in thirty-
two, a false membrane was present; most frequently, and sometimes only, on the tonsils,
sometimes on other parts also, as the palate, uvula, and pharynx. In one case no such membrane
was present; but it was found to exist in the larynx
after death. These thirty-three cases were treated
by the ordinary therapeutic measures; and of the
whole number *three* only recovered; in thirty the
disease proved fatal." It is not at all surprising
that, under these circumstances, Dr. Ware, eminent for his careful investigation and conscienti-
ous inquiry after truth, should have become "confirmed in the opinion," as he subsequently declares himself to have been, "that the methods of
treating this disease, in common use, require a
careful reconsideration;" nor, that he should

have propounded the question: "If the mode of treating croup commonly adopted, does no good, are we sure that it does no hurt?"

Having concluded after the experience to which we have referred, to treat the disease "without the persevering use of the heroic remedies," Dr. Ware subsequently adopted a method in which the treatment consisted—

1. "In the absence of all reducing, depleting, and disturbing remedies.

2. "Keeping the patient under the full influence of opium combined with calomel.

3. "Constant external application of warmth and moisture (to the neck), and of mercurial liniment, slightly stimulating.

4. "Constant inhalation of watery vapor."

In March, 1850, Dr. Ware read before the Suffolk District Medical Society "*Additional Remarks on the Treatment of Croup*," in which paper he refers to five cases of membranous croup, three of which were treated on the method indicated in the preceding propositions; and in the other two cases, in addition to these general measures, applications of a solution of nitrate of silver were made into the larynx. The first three cases which received general treatment only, proved fatal; yet they "exhibited," says Dr. Ward, "certain differences from the common course of this disease which indicated a favorable influence from difference of treatment."

"In all of them the membrane was thrown up in considerable quantities.

"In all of them the disease was attended by very much less distress than is usual in croup; and, in two, there was so decided a mitigation of symptoms following the separation of the membrane, as to lead to considerable hope of a favorable termination.

"In two, at least, the disease was prolonged to at least twice its average duration under the usual treatment.

"In the other two cases, to which reference was made, the same general course of treatment was followed, with the addition of the introduction of the sponge, wet with a solution of the nitrate of silver, into the larynx. In each of these cases the application was made as early in the disease as I became satisfied of its distinct character. It was repeated morning and evening. It decidedly gave relief to the breathing, soon after each application, and both cases ultimately recovered perfectly. For the suggestion and adoption of this valuable addition to our means of treating this formidable disease, we are indebted, as is well known, to the enterprise of Dr. Horace Green, of New York. The profession, I think, owe to him a large debt of gratitude, for the energy and perseverance manifested in the introduction of this remedy, and I am the more disposed to render this tribute to him, because so many attempts have been made to detract from his merit in relation to it.

"I am well satisfied from what I have now seen of this method of treating croup, as compared with that which has been followed for so many years, that it has the advantages which were pointed out in one of the preceding papers. It is a disease which I would treat without depletion, except, perhaps, by a few leeches—without vomiting, without purging, without blisters, without antimonials, ipecac., and all those other nauseous remedies which have been usually resorted to. I would trust to opiates, perhaps calomel, emollients, and the local application of the nitrate of silver." "I ought to add that many of my friends in the profession have informed me of cases in their practice, treated on these principles, which have recovered in a favorable manner."[1]

Since the publication of Dr. Ware's papers, cauterization of the larynx, in the treatment of membranous croup, has been adopted by large numbers of medical men in New England, as well as in other places in the United States, from many of whom we have received communications on this subject, expressing their full confidence in this therapeutic agent, when timely and appropriately employed in the management of croup.

Should we give the history of a tithe of these cases, which have been thus reported to us, they would occupy a much larger space than can be appropriated to this subject.

In 1848 the chairman of this committee published a small treatise "*On the Pathology of Croup, and its Treatment by Topical Medications,*" in which the declaration was made that "the practice of making topical applications of medicinal agents into the larynges of young children, for the treatment of membranous croup, is a plan entirely practicable, safe, and when judiciously employed, *in the highest degree efficacious.*" This method of treating a disease hitherto so unmanageable was founded, among others, upon the following propositions (which were then advanced, with regard to the pathology of the disease), namely: "that the essential characteristics of true croup consist in an inflammation of the secreting surfaces of the fauces, larynx, and trachea, which is always productive of a membranaceous or an albuminous exudation."

"2. That the membranaceous concretion, which is found coating the inflamed mucous surface of the parts in croup, is an exudation, not from the membrane itself, but is secreted by the muciparous glands, which so abundantly stud the larynx and trachea.

"3. That the exudative inflammation commences, invariably, in the superior portion of the respiratory passages, and extends from above downwards, never in the opposite direction."[1]

Since the publication of the work in which this mode of treatment is advocated, the author has had the opportunity of treating many cases of croup on the plan deduced from this view of its pathology, viz: by means of topical medication, not only in his own practice, but in the practice of, and in conjunction with, other members of the medical profession; and with an amount of success that has afforded a high degree of encouragement and satisfaction.

He has also received from medical men, in different parts of the United States, as well as from numbers in Europe, the history of many cases of membranous croup, wherein topical measures, in their hands, have proved effectual in arresting the disease.

4th. *The Effects of the Applications of the Nitrate of Silver in the Treatment of Oedema of the Glottis.*

In 1852, a work "*On the Surgical Treatment of Polypi of the Larynx, and Oedema of the Glottis,*" was published by the author, in which cases of the latter disease are reported as having been successfully treated, as early as 1849, by means of a solution of the nitrate of silver to the affected parts. The happy result which had followed its employment, encouraged the author to commend with much confidence, this method of treating one of the most formidable, and hitherto, one of the most fatal of all the diseases of the larynx.

In a paper read before the Edinburgh Medico-Chirurgical Society, by Dr. John Scott, one of the oldest and most distinguished physicians of Edinburgh—a paper which was afterwards published in the *Monthly Journal of Medical Science* for 1850—many interesting cases of laryngeal diseases, successfully treated by topical treatment, are recorded. Among the cases reported by Dr. Scott is one, the particulars of which were furnished him by his friend, Dr. Brown, of Edinburgh; which appears to have been a case of oedema of the glottis, following, or being complicated with inflammation of the mucous membrane of the parts. The patient was recovering from an attack of erysipelatous sore throat, when Dr. Brown was sent for, the message being that the patient was dying. "Meeting fortunately with Dr. Scott," says Dr. B., "he accompanied me. The patient had all the appearance of imminent death; his face expressive of extreme terror and anguish; the extremities cold; the pulse hardly to be counted from its rapidity and weakness; the breathing all but impossible, apparently from some affection at the top of the windpipe; the voice was gone. On looking deeply into the throat, the pharynx and top of the larynx were seen of a deep red.

"The patient being too weak for bloodletting, and too ill for any slower measures of relief, Dr. Scott applied the solution of the nitrate of silver, which he happened to have with him. He got the sponge completely into the larynx. Mr. S. almost instantly expressed, by signs, his relief. In the evening he could speak a little, and able to lie down in bed, and was in all respects better. He was blistered, and had calomel and opium.

"Next morning he was much better. The sponge was again applied without any difficulty. He recovered rapidly, and has been for more than two years in perfect health, attributing without any hesitation, the saving of his life to the sponge and the caustic."

The valuable work of Dr. Watson contains his views with regard to the effects of nitrate of silver in the oedematous glottis, together with a record of several cases successfully treated by this remedy; and he expresses the gratification that he has been able to "come to precisely the same conclusions with myself, as to the strength and mode of application of the solution," in the management of this disease. He therefore quotes from my work the following directions, which are to be pursued in the employment of this remedy.

"The first application with the sponge-probang should be made to the pharynx and top of the epiglottis; and after a delay of ten or fifteen minutes, the measure may be repeated, and the sponge, wet with the solution, be freely applied to the base of the epiglottis and over the oedematous lips of the glottis. The application should be repeated every hour or two hours, according to the urgency of the disease, and the effect produced by the operation; and an attempt should be made each time to carry the sponge between the lips of the glottis. As the oedema at the opening of the larynx subsides, this may be done, and the application of the caustic solution be made to the interior of the glottis.

"I am inclined to think that the benefit arising from such a practice is brought about by the powerful stimulation of the relaxed vessels of the oedematous organ. Such a condition of the bloodvessels permits a continual increase of the morbid state, whereas, by their contracting under the stimulation, the current of blood within them is quickened, and the effused fluid is partly absorbed into the circulating fluid, partly removed by the new layer of epithelium, which is rapidly found to replace what had perished during the inactivity of the basement membrane, coincident with, and produced by the oedema of its subjacent tissue. Every touch of the probang renews the impulse already given to these restorative processes, and thus the benefit increases in a geometrical ratio, till the cure is finally accomplished."[1]

"The action of a solution of caustic," says Dr. W., on another page, "applied to a sub-acutely inflamed mucous membrane, might, *a priori*, be expected to produce a beneficial effect on the oedematous glottis; and this expectation has been remarkably fulfilled in my experience."[2]

5th *Of the Effects of Nitrate of Silver in the Treatment of Hooping-Cough.*

To Professor Watson, of Glasgow, belongs the honor of having been the first to employ topical medication for the treatment of Hooping-Cough. His original paper on hooping-cough, in which he describes, "a new method of treating that disease," was read before the Medical Society of Glasgow, in 1849, and was first published in the

Edinburgh Monthly Journal in December of the
same year. Five years later—after having treated
many other cases by this new method, Dr. Watson
publishes, in his work on *Topical Medication*, the
results of his experience; and these practical results have been considered in the highest degree
encouraging. He has also given us, in this chapter
on the laryngeal treatment of hooping-cough, the
experience of *M. Joubert*, of France, who has employed, with great success, this topical method of
treatment, in a large number of cases of hooping-
cough. His memoir on the subject was published
in a French journal, in 1851.[1]

In the opinion of Dr. Watson the indications
for the topical treatment of hooping-cough are
founded upon what is considered by him the true
pathology of the disease. The morbific agent, he
thinks, whatever that poison may be, "in the cases
of hooping-cough commences its operations by
producing inflammation of the pharyngo-
laryngeal mucous membrane; and secondarily,
irritation of the pneumogastric nerves."[2] And
hence the declaration of his belief that topical
treatment alone "is founded on the true pathology of the disease, and is fitted to counteract, the
most speedily and effectually of all known means,
the results of the mysterious poison which originates the malady."[3]

In the early stage of the disease, when the inflammatory action is high, Dr. Watson recommends, for children, the employment of a solution of nitrate of silver, of the strength of about
fifteen grains to the ounce of water.

"Afterwards, when the nervous symptoms pre-
dominate, the solution may with advantage be
strengthened; but it is impossible to lay down

rules that will universally apply to different cases, or even to the same case on different days. This must be left to the judgment of the practitioner."[4] It is recommended that the applications should be made at least every second day, first to the pharyngo-laryngeal membrane, then to the parts above the glottis, and to the opening of the glottis. "But after the general inflammatory state had been got rid of," says Dr. Watson, "and when the disease has come to its height, the larynx must be entered, in order that the caustic may be brought into contact with the nerves, upon the excitement of which the continuance of the hoop depends."[1]

The following numerical account is given by Dr. Watson, of the results of the treatment in question, in his own cases, and in those of M. Joubert; the number of patients treated amounts to 134 in all:—

Cured in two weeks . . . . . . 96 cases, or   54.4 per cent
    "   three to four weeks. 61 "   or   36.5   "
Resisted treatment. 9   "
Died . . . . 1 case, or nearly 0.06   "

During the spring of 1854, hooping-cough prevailed in Glasgow as an epidemic, and Dr. Watson had an opportunity of treating a large number of cases. In the most of these the disease was very severe; and yet the result as given is as follows: cured in a fortnight *ten* cases; in three weeks *sixteen*; in four weeks *five*; *one* resisted the treatment; and *one* died.

The whole number treated being therefore 167, the proportions stand thus:—

	Cured within a fortnight	Cured within 3 or 4 weeks	Resisted treatment	Total
Dr. Watson's cases ...	46	20	0	66
M. Joubert's '' ...	40	20	8	68
	86	40	8	134

In contrast with the preceding results of the topical treatment of hooping-cough, Dr. Watson subjoins a table of the ordinary duration of the disease when treated in the usual manner, as stated by some of the best and most recent authorities, such as Williams, Copland, Walsh, West, and a few others; and the average of all the statements of these authors, is from one and a half to three and a half months.

The deaths from hooping-cough in London (and the percentage appears to be about the same in other parts of Great Britain), according to the reports of the Registrar-General, are in the proportion of 8.9 per cent among females, and 6.2 per cent among males to the deaths from all causes under ten years of age.

"Surely, then," adds Prof. Watson, "a treatment which promised to diminish, or perhaps to annihilate this great mortality, ought to have been received with consideration by the profession," for, as the author subsequently remarks, "the numerical results just given prove in a manner beyond all cavil, that the simple treatment which I have suggested is capable of cutting short the hooping-cough with as much certainty as quinine arrests an intermittent fever; and

moreover, that it renders the disease while it lasts
both milder in type, and safer to the patient than
the most favorable circumstances of season or
epidemic could possibly do."[1]

So far as your committee has been able to learn,
it is ascertained that this topical method for the
treatment of hooping-cough has been employed
only to a very limited extent in this country. During the last four years every case of hooping-
cough which has occurred in the practice of the
chairman of your Committee (and they amount
to a considerable number of cases), has been
treated by applications of a solution of nitrate of
silver to the pharyngo-laryngeal mucous membrane. In all these instances, the peculiar symptoms of the disease, the spasmodic cough and
hoop, have been arrested in from one to two
weeks; and in several cases which occurred last
winter, the hoop ceased entirely after the third
application of the remedy: the cough, also, disappeared in a short time after. So far, then, as the
experience of your Committee goes, it substan-
tiates fully the favorable results obtained by Watson and Joubert.

Although to Dr. Watson has been awarded the
honor of being the first who employed topical
medication for the treatment of hooping-cough,
still it would seem to be not inappropriate here to
explain, as Dr. Watson has himself done, with
great candor and fairness, "the way by which he
came to try" this method of topical applications
for the treatment of the disease in question.
"Soon after the publication of Dr. Horace Green's
work on *Diseases of the Air-passages*, he observes,
"I had several opportunities of putting to the test
of experience his method of treating chronic

laryngeal affections, viz: by touching the lining of
the larynx with a solution of the nitrate of silver.
My trials fully confirmed his statement of the
efficacy of the treatment referred to, and I soon
found that I could with advantage carry out a
similar practice in many other diseases, such as in
ordinary acute bronchitis, in the intervals of asthma, and even with relief of the tickling cough in
early phthisis. Having thus established, to my satisfaction, the efficacy of a topical application of
caustic solution in cases not only of chronic disease of the larynx but in all cases of inflammatory
irritation of the glottis, I came to the conclusion
that it might operate beneficially in the hooping-
cough; and, after a pretty extensive trial, I have
not been disappointed."[1]

In closing this interesting chapter on topical
medication, in hooping-cough, Dr. Watson expresses the hope that the day is not distant when
the treatment, "so well described by these excellent writers, and the usefulness of which," he says,
"I have now been enabled to establish, not only by
its results in my own practice but also in that of M.
Joubert, will be more favorably received in this
country, and more generally adopted by British
practitioners of medicine;" a hope which, by my
own experience, I have been led most sincerely to
entertain with regard to the practitioners of my
own country.

6th. *Of the Effects of Nitrate of Silver in the Treatment of Spasmodic Asthma.*
If the histological observations of some recent
pathologists be correct with regard to the nature
of spasmodic asthma, it might be anticipated, *a
priori*, that the application of a solution of nitrate

of silver to the affected parts, would produce a most beneficial effect on the disease; and so far these expectations, in the experience of all those who have tried this remedy, have been entirely fulfilled. It is well known that there are only certain points in the course of the air-tubes at which a spasm can occur sufficient to produce the dyspnoea that takes place in asthma, and these portions are where the contraction of muscular fibres is not prevented by the existence of cartilaginous rings; the principal points are at the extremities of the bronchial tubes, and at the rima glottidis. Williams, in his work on the *Pathology and Diagnosis of Diseases of the Chest,* expresses the opinion that the contraction of the former, "the bronchial muscles, is a sufficient cause of spasmodic asthma."[2] Dr. Hastings believes that the constriction occurs in the larynx,[3] and Dr. Watson declares that the constriction in the minute bronchi cannot satisfactorily explain the complete stoppage of the breathing which occurs in the paroxysm. For this it seems absolutely necessary to assume that closure of the glottis likewise takes place on these occasions.[1]

Founded on these views of the nature of this disease, the last two named authors have adopted the plan of topical medication, in spasmodic asthma, and this treatment in their hands has been attended with complete success.

"In spasmodic asthma," Dr. Hastings remarks, "percussion elicits a tolerably clear sound from the thoracic walls. On applying the ear or the stethoscope below the clavicles, sibilant and sonorous rattles are heard. These diminish as we proceed in the examination towards the abdomen, but increase as we pass upwards towards the neck, and over the trachea or larynx their greatest intensity is evident, which region is, moreover, the real seat of the disease. The sounds heard in the chest are transmitted from this part, and this fact admits of ready demonstration.

"If a sponge soaked in a solution of the nitrate of silver be passed over the diseased surface, and the chest be examined immediately afterwards, the sibilant and sonorous rattles will have partially or entirely disappeared, and those of the laryngeal region become so much diminished that they cannot be propagated into the tubes within the lungs. Yet how repeatedly have I seen such patients with their chests cupped, leeched and blistered!"[2]

Several interesting cases of this disease are recorded by Dr. Hastings as having been successfully treated by topical medication. In one instance, the applications of a solution of the nitrate of silver failed to effect a cure when the author substituted a saturated solution of the bicyanuret of mercury in distilled water, under the use of which, and of light tonics, combined with nitric acid, the patient rapidly improved, and was restored to permanent health.[3]

"The state of the larynx," says Dr. Watson, "in spasmodic asthma, has not hitherto received adequate attention either from pathologists or physicians; in this opinion he expresses himself fully confirmed, that a morbid contraction of the larynx is a frequent cause of the disease, and that a spasm of the glottis dependent upon a lesion of this organ, constitutes an essential part of a fit of asthma.

On the subject of the treatment of this disease by local measures, Dr. Watson remarks: "I am far

from wishing to laud the topical applications beyond what they deserve, but I am sure any medical
practitioner will bear me out in saying, that the
ordinary treatment of asthma, by bleeding, general or local, by emetics, antispasmodics, opiates,
and mercurials internally, with blisters and various other counter-irritants externally, has seldom
been followed by even a partial success in these
cases." "There is here, therefore, an evident
blank in therapeutics, for no agent hitherto proposed has been found capable (says Dr. W.) of
removing or greatly diminishing this morbid contractility of the air-tubes."[1] A solution of caustic,
in the opinion of the author, "applied to the interior of the larynx, supplies this defect, fills up
the blank." And he has recorded in his work
many severe cases of spasmodic asthma, successfully treated, in the management of which no
other means were employed, "but the regular
application of caustic to the affected parts, at first
every day, and afterwards every second day."[2] In
the last edition of my work on "*Diseases of the Air-
Passages*", several cases of spasmodic asthma are
recorded, in the treatment of which cauterizations were employed with entire success; it has
been, therefore, a cause of gratulation, that the
statements of your Committee, with respect to the
efficacy of the treatment have been fully confirmed in the experience of these distinguished practitioners.

Since we commenced drawing up this report, a
new work, *On the Local Treatment of the Mucous
Membrane of the Throat, for Cough and Bronchitis*,
recently published in London, by J.E. Riadore,
has been received. This work, in which topical
medication for the treatment of many affections

of the air-passages is advocated, contains nothing
particularly new or important on this subject.
The only novel suggestion made by the author, is
one respecting the *temperature* of the solutions to
be employed in local treatment. In spasmodic
asthma, particularly, the author urges the employment of a *hot* solution of nitrate of silver.
Indeed, he advises that, in all spasmodic cases of
the organs of the throat, the remedial ap-
pliances—the solutions, should be made hot, and
used as warm as they can be borne."[3]

7th. *Of the Effects of Nitrate of Silver employed as a
Topical Remedy in the Treatment of Tuberculosis,
following or complicated with Bronchial Inflammation.*

Ten years ago, in 1846, in a work to which I
have before alluded (*On Diseases of the Air-Passages*), topical applications of the nitrate of silver
were recommended to be employed in the treatment of Tuberculosis. On page 260 of this work is
the following declaration: "Among the cases of
laryngeal and bronchial affection, which, during
the year 1845, came under my care, twenty-five
presented decided symptoms of pulmonary
phthisis, complicated with follicular disease. As
the pulmonary symptoms, in a majority of the
cases, had supervened upon the original glandu-
lar affection, topical measures were employed—
not with the expectation of their proving ultimately remedial, but with the hope of deferring
the pulmonary, by allaying the laryngeal disease;
and the success which has attended these efforts
in a majority of the above cases, in mitigating the
sufferings and in prolonging the lives of my pa-

tients, has been to me a source of the highest gratification."

This proposition to treat a general disease by local measures, was not at that time, received with favor by the medical profession. And yet, the plan has since been adopted by large numbers of the intelligent portion of the profession in our own, and in foreign countries, who have given the highest testimony in its favor. Not only is laryngeal inflammation present in varying degrees of intensity in the early period of tuberculosis, but recent histological observations have fully established this pathological fact, that in all cases of tubercular deposit, there occurs in the immediate vicinity of the exudation more or less of an inflammatory action, in which all the adjacent structures are involved. The bronchial membrane and the pulmonary parenchyma become at once congested, and subsequently inflamed. The terminal extremities of the bronchi, says Prof. Bennett, are among the first structures affected, and as the tuberculosis proceeds, all the appearances characteristic of chronic bronchitis are produced, and are constantly going on in the progress of a case. "consequently," he observes, "the great problem to be worked out, in the treatment of pulmonary tuberculosis, is that while, on the one hand, it is a disease of diminished nutrition and weakness, and consequently requires a general invigorating and supporting system of treatment, on the other, it is accompanied by local excitement, which demands an antiphlogistic and lowering practice."[1]

It is to meet this last indication, to subdue the local inflammatory action in the immediate vicini-

ty of the exudation—an action which, if continued, will not only effectually prevent the disin-
tegration and absorption of the tubercular mass
already formed, but which will tend to augment
the mass—that applications of the nitrate of silver
solution to the congested and inflamed membrane, are advised in early, as well as in advanced
tuberculosis.

Dr. Hastings, in his *Treatise on Diseases of the
Larynx and Trachea*, has devoted a chapter to the
subject of the topical treatment of tubercular,
when complicated with laryngeal disease. In the
earliest stage of this affection, "it should be met,"
says Dr. Hastings,"by the most vigorous treatment, and I know of no means so capable of
arresting or removing it, as sponging the windpipe with a solution of the nitrate of silver."[1] Several cases are narrated by this author, which were
successfully treated by this plan, one of which, as
it is that of a surgeon of the army, and is of great
interest, I shall take the liberty of giving, ab-
breviated. This surgeon "returned from India,
in1846, on sick certificate, having suffered for
about two years previously from pulmonary disease. On leaving India, the symptoms were as
follows: Cough, with copious muco-purulent expectoration, occasionally mixed with blood; frequent pain in the upper portion of the left chest,
increased on deep inspiration; much prostration
of strength, and considerable emaciation."[2]

After his return home he improved somewhat
in health and strength, up to October, 1847,
when he was suddenly attacked with acute inflammation of the left lung. From this attack he
gradually recovered sufficiently to go to London,
in 1848, for the purpose of consulting Dr. Hast-

ings. About a week after his arrival he was again attacked with acute inflammation of the lungs, in which the larynx and trachea were involved. "At the commencement of this attack," says the patient himself, "the symptoms were as follows: Pains in the clavicular portion of the left side of the thorax, extending downwards; hurried and difficult respiration; inability to expand the chest, almost in the slightest degree, also when lying on the left side and back; quick pulse; much prostration of strength and extreme emaciation. I derived the greatest and almost immediate relief, when suffering from difficulty of breathing, from having the larynx and trachea sponged with a solution of the nitrate of silver. This attack gradually yielded to the treatment employed, when I was put on a course of the pyroacetic spirit, and cod-liver oil.

"This treatment has been continued at intervals ever since, and to which I may attribute my restoration to my present state of health."

Dr. Hastings adds: 'The writer of the above was, when he consulted me, about two years and a half ago, under forty years of age, and weighed 10 st. 6 lbs.; he now weighs 11 st. 4 lbs. When I first saw him, he had a large gurgling cavity in the upper lobe of the left lung; two or three of his medical friends laughed at the bare idea that any substantial good could be done for him. After completely removing the inflammation in the larynx and trachea, by sponging that passage twice a week with a solution of the nitrate of silver for three months, the disease in the lungs appeared gradually and steadily to diminish; and although at Christmas last, and for some time previous, he had lost all the general symptoms of phthisis, the cavity, which then was dry, and much smaller, was, however, still very evident. But now it has entirely disappeared—slight bronchophony is heard over its former seat, and more or less imperfect respiratory murmur exists in the upper portion of the lung, with considerable flattening of the superior part of the left chest."****

"My object for inserting this case here is for the purpose of showing the great advantage to be derived from sponging the laryngo-tracheal tube with the nitrate of silver, in the early stage of tubercular laryngitis."[1]

Still more extensively has Prof. Watson considered this subject; the employment of local treatment in tuberculosis; and he has recorded several most instructive cases, in which the larynx was advantageously treated by topical means, in both incipient and advanced pulmonary phthisis.

In combination with, or to be followed by appropriate general remedies, he urges the importance of the use of applications of nitrate of silver to the larynx, in all those incipient cases of phthisis in which the cough is caused by actual laryngitis, by the irritation produced by the passage of bloody sputum; or by secondary nervous irritation of the larynx. The cough in these cases, he declares, "is not simply a symptom in the ordinary acceptation of the term; it is itself a disease, the result of organic change in the larynx, which increases the pulmonary affection. In treating the larynx, therefore, with a view of diminishing the cough, the physician is not to be looked upon as irrational, but on the contrary, as aiming his remedial measures at the very source of much of the distress of the patient and of the fatal progress of the disease."[1]

No unprejudiced person can read the testimony embodied in the cases reported by Dr. Watson, without having the conviction forced upon him, that in many of these instances of early tuberculosis an arrestment of the pulmonary disease was brought about by the measures adopted. Not that the author would represent these cases as positively cured, "for undoubtedly," he remarks, "the tendency to tubercular disease still remains in the constitution, though its local manifestation has ceased to exist." * * "Formerly," he continues, "there was positive evidence of an actual consumption; now, there is no such evidence, but on the contrary, all the signs and symptoms of perfect health."[2] Some may doubt the relation of the topical treatment to the successful issue in these cases, says Dr. Watson, but no one can fail to perceive, "that the cough first abated as the laryngeal iritability was removed, then the general health improved, and *some time afterwards*, the pulmonary condensation was found to have disappeared."[3]

In the advanced stage of phthisis, in which the cough is caused or aggravated by laryngeal ulcers; or, in which the passage of purulent sputum produces laryngeal irritation, topical applications, says Dr. Watson, although they cannot be considered in the light of *curative* means, "ought nevertheless to be practiced whenever the patient can bear them, as the surest and best means of relieving him from the pain and distress which are caused by the state of the larynx; and when cautiously pursued, even in such cases, I have known more than one life prolonged for months and even years."[3]

Dr. Cotton also, in his work on consumption,

recommends the topical application of nitrate of silver to the larynx, especially in the early stage of the disease. "I would not advise it to be practiced, however," says Dr. Cotton, "when the pulmonary disease is in a *very* advanced stage, and the strength of the patient much exhausted." Its use by him is restricted to the early period of the disease, when the lungs are not much affected, not the strength of the patient reduced; it is this stage, he says, which presents the most promising opportunities for its employment.

The testimony of Dr. A. Scott Alison, in his treatise on the *Medication of the Larynx and Trachea*, is decidedly in favor of the employment of the nitrate of silver, in the treatment of that cough and irritation of the glottis, which are dependent upon the presence of tubercles in the lung. "Much comfort and benefit," he says, "have been derived from its use, both when the tubercles have been crude, and when they have become softened. The presence of undoubted cavities in the lungs, the breaking down of tubercles, and the expulsion of their debris, have not prevented this application from being decidedly useful."[1]

Prof. Robert B. Todd, Physician to King's College Hospital, London, who has had much experience, in the treatment of pharyngo-laryngeal and bronchial diseases, by topical medication, has embodied in his "Clinical Lectures," recently published in the *London Medical Times and Gazette*,[2] some of his views, and recorded his experience in relation to this subject. In the treatment of these affections, he employs and recommends "the local application of a solution of nitrate of silver (   ), by means of a probang thrust behind the epiglottis down to the glottis, on the

plan of Dr. Horace Green, of New York." "The
patient," he says, "can always tell whether the
sponge enters the larynx or not, from the great
irritation it excites when it passes into the glottis;
and in the withdrawal of it, the operator feels a
certain resistance caused by the sponge being
grasped by the muscles of the larynx, which resistance is not felt when it simply passes into the
oesophagus."[3] In one case reported by Dr. Todd,
in which the symptoms indicated confirmed
tubercular disease of the lungs, complicated with
chronic thickening of the mucous membrane of
the larynx and epiglottis, with ulceration of the
chordae vocales, and of the ventricles of the
larynx, applications of a strong solution of nitrate
of silver to the diseased parts, tended invariably
greatly to relieve the extreme irritability of the
larynx, for "the patient always expressed herself
as much better after each application, and her
pain was relieved, although only temporarily."
But in the milder forms of the disease, the topical
treatment often proved permanently beneficial;
for Dr. Todd assures us, that he "could tell of
numerous instances of coughs of the most troublesome kind, and of long duration, that had
resisted all the ordinary cough medicines, and
which had yielded to three or four applications of
the nitrate of silver."

Persons laboring under such symptoms as
these, he declares, are often treated for
bronchitis, and take large quantities of expector-
ant and other medicines, for the relief of the
cough. The seat of the irritation, upon which the
cough depends, is thought to be in the bronchial
tubes, and its real position (the fauces) is overlooked.[1]

I have already alluded to the experience of

Prof. Bennett, of Edinburgh, in the use of local applications for the treatment of those laryngeal diseases which, he assures us, are frequently mistaken for, or associated with, pulmonary tuberculosis. Dr. Bennett closes his valuable work on the pathology and treatment of pulmonary tuberculosis by the following practical conclusions:—

"1st. That not unfrequently diseases, entirely seated in the larynx or pharynx, are mistaken for pulmonary tuberculosis.

"2d. That even when pulmonary tuberculosis exists, many of the urgent symptoms are not so much owing to disease in the lung, as to the pharyngeal and laryngeal complications.

"3d. That a local treatment may not only remove or alleviate these complications, but that, in conjunction with general remedies, it tends in a marked manner to induce arrestment of the pulmonary disease."[2]

And here, the duty of the commission appointed to report to this Association "on the use and effect of applications of nitrate of silver to the throat," may be considered as fulfilled, and their work accomplished.

It was our intention, however, to have illustrated the great value of this therapeutic agent, in the treatment of the different forms of disease, to which we have referred by the history of cases which have fallen under our own observation, which would have corroborated fully the favorable reports made by the preceding authors. But this paper is already sufficiently extended. Justice to this subject, however, would not be done, should we fail to allude altogether to the success, which, during the last eighteen months, has at-

tended the still farther extension of topical medication, in the treatment of thoracic disease, effected by means of the operation of *catheterism* of
the air-passages, or the injections of a solution of
the nitrate of silver into the bronchial divisions.

During the last eighteen months, or since October, 1854, over one hundred patients, embracing cases of both pulmonary and bronchial disease, have been treated by this form of topical
medication, conjoined with appropriate general
remedies. The history of this plan of treatment
and the results which have been in a high degree
satisfactory, have been brought before the profession in papers read before the New York
Academy of Medicine; before the State Medical
Society of New York; and, more recently, a detailed report, embracing a statistical table of one
hundred and six cases, thus treated, was published in the pages of the *American Medical Monthly*.
Besides their publication in this country, most of
these papers have been reprinted in some of the
medical publications of Great Britain, and have
also been translated and republished in a few of
the leading journals of France. It will therefore
be unnecessary to bring the whole subject before
the Association; and we shall close the present
report by a brief analysis of the cases embraced in
the statistical table, which, with the history of
many of these cases, may be found in the *American Medical Monthly* for March, 1856.

Of one hundred cases of thoracic disease
treated by catheterism of the air-passages, seven-
ty-one of the sum total are recorded as cases of
tuberculosis. Of this number, *thirty-two* were considered cases of *advanced phthisis*—cases in which
tubercular cavities were recognized in one or

both lungs; and *thirty-nine* cases of *early phthisis*. Of the first division—advanced phthisis—fourteen have since died. *Twenty-five* were more or less improved; their lives being apparently prolonged by this method of medication. *Seven* only of the thirty-two cases of advanced phthisis were not benefited by the injections.

Of the *thirty-nine* cases of incipient tuberculosis, twelve of this disease have apparently recovered. Five more of this number are now, or were, at the time of making the report, in the enjoyment of a good degree of health. With respect to the above twelve cases, I say *apparently* cured; for, although the appearance of these patients, as manifested both by the physical and rational signs, is indicative of an ordinary degree of health, yet in a disease like that of tuberculosis, every medical man is aware that one year is a period too brief to speak decidedly with regard to the positive and final result.

Of the remaining *twenty-two* cases, many of whom, at the time of the report, were still under treatment, *seventeen* had been greatly improved by topical medication; three more had been moderately benefited; while *three* only had failed to obtain any advantage from the local measures which had been adopted.

Of the *twenty-eight* cases of *bronchitis*, sixteen had been dismissed, cured, or so much improved as to require no further treatment. All the others had been greatly benefited, although some were still under treatment at the time of making the report.

Finally, in view of all that has been accomplished by topical medication, the chairman of the committee would reiterate the declaration made in the first paper communicated to the professional public on this subject, that, "the results of this method of treating disease, whether it has been employed in bronchial affections, or in the commencement of tuberculosis, have already afforded the most gratifying indications that practical medicine will be greatly advanced by this discovery."[1]

HORACE GREEN.

NOTES

[1]The Topical Medication of the Larynx in Certain Diseases of the Respiratory and Vocal Organs. By Eben Watson, A.M, M.D.&c.&c.

[2]Op. citat., p.32

[3]Op. citat.,pp. 32-3.

[4]The Pathology and Treatment of Pulmonary Tuberculosis; and on the Local Medication of Pharyngeal and Laryngeal Diseases, frequently mistaken for, or associated with, Phthisis. By John Hughes Bennett, M.D., F.R.S.E., &c.&c., p.140.

[5]The Medication of the Larynx and Trachea. By S. Scott Alison, M.D., &c., pp. 10,11.

[6]A Treatise on Diseases of the Air-Passages, &c., p.213.

[7]Op. citat., p. 128.

[8]A Treatise on Diseases of the Larynx and Trachea. By John Hastings, M.D., &c. London, pp.115.

[9]Op. Citat., pp. 116-7.

[10]Op. citat., p. 119

[11]Ib., pp. 139,140.

[12]Op. Citat., pp. 236-7.

[13]Op. citat., pp. 79,80,81.

[14]Ib., p. 85 et seq.

[15]Ib., p. 130.

[16]Op. citat., p.40.

[17]Ib., p.41.

[18]Op. citat., p. 41.

[19]Ib., p.140.

[20]Ib., p. 85 et seq.

[21]Op. citat., pp. 23.

[22]Ib., pp.7 and 8.

[23]American Medical Monthly, Jan. 1855, p.9.

[24]See American Med. Monthly, pp. 9-10.
[25]Manuel Pratique des Maladies des Nouveaux-Nés, et des Enfants à la Mamelle, p. 272.
[26]Archives Générales de Medecine, tome xix., art. 1st.
[27]The only other case mentioned by Dr. Watson, as one not benefited by the topical treatment, is that of a gentleman past the middle period of life, "who on a winter evening," was suddenly seized with difficult respiration, tightness in the throat, harsh, dry, whistling cough, and high fever, "whilst the physical signs were: Inspiration long in the trachea, and accompanied by a harsh sound of the air passing along the dry and narrowed tube." Symptoms, manifestly indicative of *acute laryngitis*, and not as Dr. Watson supposed, of "ACUTE TRACHEAL CROUP, accompanied by exudation."*
*Op. citat., p. 51.
[28]Op. citat., pp. 49,50.
[29]Op. citat., pp. 51,52.
[30]Ib., p. 51.
[31]Boston Med. and Surgical Journal, vol. xlii. pp. 267-8.
[32]Observations on the Pathology of Croup, with Remarks on its Treatment by Topical Medications, &c.
[33]Watson, pp. 57,58.
[34]Ib., pp.54,55.
[35]Recueil des Travaux de la Société Médicale de l'Indre et Loire. 1851.
[36]Op. citat., p. 107.
[37]Ib., p. 106.
[38] Ib., p. 116.
[39]Op. citat., p. 118.
[40]Op. citat., p. 124.
[41]Monthly Journal of Medical Sciences, Dec., 1849, p. 1290.
[42]Pathology and Diagnosis of Diseases of the Chest, &c., p. 91.
[43]Op. citat., p. 66.
[44]Op. citat., p. 127.
[45]Ib., p.66.
[46]Ib., pp. 68-9.
[47]Op. citat., pp. 134-6.
[48]Ib., p. 132.
[49]Ut supra, p.96.
[50]Op. citat., p. 68.
[51]Op. citat., p. 130.
[52]Ib., p. 130.
[53]Op. citat., pp. 131-133.
[54]Op. citat., p. 168.
[55]Ib., p. 172.
[56]Ib., p. 180.
[56]Medication of the Larynx and Trachea, &c., p. 8.

[58]Medical Times and Gazette, No. 139, p.207.
[59]Ib., p. 210.
[60]Op. citat., p. 209.
[61]Ib., p. 142.
[62]American Medical Monthly, Jan. 1855, p.25.

THE TREATMENT OF ACUTE RHEUMATISM BY SALICIN.

By T. MACLAGAN, M.D.

Reprinted from LANCET *1:342-3, 383-4, 1876*

Perusal of the literature which bears on the question of the treatment of acute rheumatism is a task from which few would rise with any definite idea as to how that disease is best treated. Purgatives, diaphoretics, sedatives, alkalies and alkaline salts, colchicum, aconite, quinine, guaiacum, lemon-juice, sulphur, mercury, veratria, tincture of muriate of iron, &c., would each be found to have in turn attracted the favourable notice of one or more of those who have directed attention to the subject. Of all these different remedies, not one stands out prominently as that to which we can with confidence look for good results. "Each and every plan of treatment which has been hitherto proposed is regarded by the profession as unsatisfactory."* In accordance with this impression, we find eminent and trustworthy physicians treating the disease on a purely expectant plan—that is, not giving drugs at all, and apparently with results as satisfactory as those which follow the administration of any of the usual remedies.† We have, indeed, no remedy for acute rheumatism—a malady which not unfrequently proves fatal, which is always accompanied by great pain, and is a fruitful source of heart disease.

Under these circumstances, I need make no apology for bringing under the notice of the profession a remedy which, so far as my observations have gone, has given better results than which I have hitherto tried, and I have tried all the usual remedies over and over again.

In the course of an investigation into the causation and pathology of acute febrile ailments, which has for some time engaged my attention, I was led to give some consideration to intermittent and to rheumatic fever. The more I studied these ailments the more was I struck with the points of analogy which existed between them. On a detailed consideration of these I shall not now enter. Suffice it to say that they were sufficiently marked to lead me to regard rheumatic fever as being, in its pathology, more closely allied to intermittent fever than to any other disease, an opinion which further reflection and extended experience have served only to strengthen.

Rheumatic fever is now-a-days generally regarded as being produced by some cause or agency which is generated within the body. My own investigations into its pathology have led me to reject this view, and to adopt the old "miasmatic" view of its mode of origin, according to which the cause which gives rise to the disease is introduced into the system from without.

Holding this view as to the pathology of rheumatic fever, impressed with the points of resemblance between it and intermittant fever, and bearing in mind that we have in quinine a potent remedy against the latter, there seemed to me good reason for indulging the hope that some remedy would yet be discovered capable of exercising a similar, if not equally beneficial action on rheumatic fever.

In reference to the action of quinine on the various forms of intermittent and remittent fever, and, indeed, with reference to the action of the Chinchonaceae generally on the diseases of tropical climates (ipecacuanha in dysentery, for instance), there is one fact which has always strongly impressed me—the fact, namely, that the maladies on whose course they exercise the most beneficial action are most prevalent in those countries in which the Chinchonaceae grow most readily; nature seeming to produce the remedy under climatic conditions similar to those which give rise to the disease. Impressed with this fact, and believing in the miasmatic origin of rheumatic fever, it seemed to me that a remedy for that disease would most hopefully be looked for among those plants and trees whose favourite habitat presented conditions analogous to those under which the rheumatic miasm seemed most to prevail. A low-lying, damp locality, with a cold, rather than warm, climate, give the conditions under which rheumatic fever is most readily produced. On reflection, it seemed to me that the plants whose haunts best corresponded to such a description were those belonging to the natural order Salicaceae, the various forms of willow. Among the Salicaceae, therefore, I determined to search for a remedy for acute rheumatism. The bark of many species of willow contains a bitter principle called salicin. This principle was exactly what I wanted: to it, therefore, I determined to

have recourse. It will thus be seen that the employment of salicin in the treatment of acute
rheumatism was no haphazard experiment, but
had a fair foundation in reason and analogy.

Salicin has long enjoyed a reputation for tonic
and febrifuge properties, and was at one time a
good deal used as a substitute for quinine. It has
of late years, however, gone very much out of use,
and now it does not even find a place in the
British Pharmacopoeia.

The idea of treating acute rheumatism by salicin occurred to me in November, 1874. I had at
the time under my care a well-marked case of the
disease (Case 1) which was being treated by alkalies, but was not improving. I determined to
give salicin; but before doing so, took myself first
five, then ten, and then thirty grains without experiencing the least inconvenience or discomfort.
Satisfied as to the safety of its administration, I
gave to the patient referred to twelve grains every
three hours. The result exceeded my most san-
guine expectations. For some days prior to its
administration the temperature had ranged from
101.8° to 103°; the pulse was 120, and the joints
were swollen and very painful. On the 26th of
November the alkaline treatment was stopped,
and that by salicia commenced. On the following
day, after eighty-four grains of salicin had been
taken, the pulse had gone down to 100, the temperature to 99.6° (from 102.8° the previous day),
a fall of over 3°, the pain and swelling of joints,
but especially the pain, had much abated, the
joints could be moved a little, and the patient
expressed himself as being much better. On the
next day (Nov. 28th) the temperature was natural
and the pain all but gone, the joints still remain-

ing stiff. From this time he convalesced steadily and quickly.

The case was a very striking one; but, by itself, could not be regarded as proof of the beneficial action of salicin. I was quite aware that cases of acute rheumatism do sometimes unexpectedly improve without any treatment, and had no surety that this was not a case in point. It afforded me, however, strong encouragement to persevere with the salicin. This I did; and all the cases of acute and sub-acute, and several of the cases of chronic, rheumatism which have come under my care since then have been treated by this remedy, and with results much more satisfactory than I ever got from any other remedy,—the results being most marked and most satisfactory in distinctly acute cases, and least so in chronic cases. Subjoined are the details of eight cases; four acute, three subacute, and one chronic.

CASE 1. *Acute rheumatism*—William R——, aged forty-eight, was first seen on Nov. 24th, 1874. Had rheumatic fever eight years ago; was then confined to bed for eight weeks. With that exception has always enjoyed good health. Present illness commenced three days ago with shivering and pains in joints, which have increased in severity.

Nov. 24th.—Has anxious, pained expression. Lies on his back without power of motion, the least movement causing intense pain. Skin covered with acid perspiration; tongue moist and furred; bowels moved by medicine; urine scanty and high-coloured; pulse 120, small and regular; temperature 101.8°; heart's sounds normal. To have twenty grains of acetate of potass every four hours, and ten grains of Dover's powder at bed-time. Food to consist of milk, beef-tea, and light puddings.

25th.—Passed an almost sleepless night. General state unchanged. Has great pain in the joints, especially in the knees, ankles, wrists, and fingers, which are all a good deal swollen. Cannot move. Pulse 120, feeble; temperature 103°; heart's sounds a little muffled; skin bathed in acid perspiration. Continue treatment.

26th.—Had an hour's troubled sleep after the Dover's powder. No change in general condition; lies on his back, quite unable to move; profuse perspiration; pulse 120, feeble; heart-sounds indistinct; temperature 102.8°. Omit potass and Dover's powder; to have twelve grains of salicin every three hours.

27th.—Had four powders (forty-eight grains) before bedtime yesterday. Passed a much better night; slept for several hours in snatches of an hour at a time. Expresses himself as feeling much better, and looks so; says the powders did him a deal of good; can move his limbs a little, but not without pain; joints less swollen; skin covered with acid perspiration; tongue furred; bowels not moved; pulse 100, of better volume, soft and compressible; heart-sounds clearer; temperature 99.6°. Has had eighty-four grains of salicin. To continue it.

28th.—Had a pretty good night; pain nearly gone, though still felt on moving the limbs; joints almost natural in size, except those of the fingers, which are still swollen; skin not perspiring so freely; secretion still acid; tongue cleaning; bowels not moved. Pulse 84, of good volume and character; heart-sounds distinct and normal;

temperature 98 5°. To have a dose of castor oil, and to continue salicin every four hours.

29th.—Passed a good night; pains quite gone, and can move the joints freely. Is loud in his praise of the powders, every one of which, he says, he felt do him good; wishes to continue them. Pulse 72; temperature 98.3°.

From this time convalescence was steady and satisfactory.

CASE 2. *Acute rheumatism*.—Mrs. B——, aged thirty-three. First seen on Dec. 18th, 1874. On Dec. 15th was seized with pains in hips and knees, for which she was compelled to go to bed. Had been shivering and feeling out of sorts for two or three days before.

Dec. 18th.—Complains of pain in both knees, and in left wrist, which are all swollen and tender; skin covered with acid perspiration; tongue furred; bowels moved by medicine; urine scanty and high-coloured; pulse 116; temperature 101.6°. To have twelve grains of salicin every four hours.

19th.—Not much sleep; general condition unchanged. Pulse 116; temperature 102.2°. To take a powder every three hours.

20th.—Better night; feels much better; can move knees without pain, though joints are still stiff; is quite free from pain; tongue cleaner; skin moist. Pulse 84; temperature 99°.

21st.—Feels quite well; only a little stiff. Pulse 72; temperature 98.5°.

Convalesced satisfactorily.

CASE 3. *Acute rheumatism*.—Henry B——, aged thirty-four, had rheumatic fever seven years ago; was ill at that time for six or seven weeks.

March 14th.—Two days ago felt generally out of sorts; at night felt cold and shivering and had aching pains in limbs, especially in hip joints. Complains now of pain in right shoulder, both ankles, and left knee, the ankles and shoulder being most painful; all the affected joints are slightly swollen. Feels just as he did when his fever came on seven years ago. Has anxious expression; skin covered with acid perspiration; tongue thickly furred; bowels moved by medicine. Pulse 112; temperature 102.1°; heart's sounds normal. To have twenty grains of salicin every three hours.

15th.—Rather restless night; ankles and shoulder not so painful, but left knee more so; through some mistake did not have the powders during the night; free acid perspiration; pulse 120; temperature 101°. Continue salicin; heart's sounds normal.—Evening: Feels better; says the powders are giving him much relief. Pulse 100; temperature 99.3°. Continue salicin.

16th.—Passed a much better night; skin moist; tongue less furred; expression much improved. Pulse 80; temperature 98.6° All the joints free from pain, though stiff and giving slight pain on motion.

17th.—Feels quite well. Pulse 68; temperature 98.2°.

CASE 4. *Acute rheumatism.*—J. G——, aged twenty-six. On Feb. 8th was ailing, and at night was siezed with severe pain in the back and limbs, accompanied by fever and tenderness of painful parts.

Feb. 9th.—Skin hot and covered with acid perspiration; tongue furred; bowels moved; has great pain in lumbar region, in knees, in calves of legs, and in elbow and wrist joints, all which parts are tender on pressure; no headache; pulse 104; temperature 102.5°. To have fifteen grains of salicin every two hours.

10th.—Had a better night; pain much less; feels that the powders do him good; tongue cleaner; profuse acid perspiration; bowels moved; pulse 100 temperature 99.5°.

11th.—Passed a good night; is almost free from pain; still perspiring freely; pulse 70; temperature 98.3°.

Remained well, except for aching in knees for a few days.

CASE 5. *Subacute rheumatism.*—Jane S——, aged twenty-three. For the last three weeks has had rheumatic pains, for which she has been taking nitrate of potass with some benefit.

Nov. 30th.—Five days ago she had shivering and much increase of pain. Face flushed; skin warm, not perspiring; pulse 108; temperature 100.8°; heart normal; tongue furred in centre; the joints of wrists and fingers are swollen and tender on both hands; knees psinful and tender to touch, but not swollen. To have half an ounce of castor oil, and twenty grains of salicin every four hours.

Dec. 1st.—No salicin to be had from chemist; has therefore had none. Bowels acted; passed a restless night; had a good deal of pain; wrists and fingers still much swollen; pulse 92; temperature 100°.

2nd.—Commenced the salicin yesterday evening; had rather a restless night; general state much the same; pulse 96; temperature 100.3°.

3rd.—Passed a much better night; pains gone from wrists and knees, but has a little pain in left shoulder, which is tender to the touch; fingers and wrists can now be freely moved without pain; pulse 76; temperature 98.6°.

Progressed favourably.

CASE 6. *Subacute rheumatism*.—William M——, aged thirty, has twice had rheumatic fever. Is of nervous temperament.

Dec. 28th.—For the last two or three days he has felt generally out of sorts, and has had pain in left knee, which has also been swollen. Slept badly last night, and to-day feels general sense of discomfort; has pain in left knee, in both ankles, and to some extent in shoulders; the right ankle and left knee are swollen and tender to the touch; skin natural; tongue slightly furred; pulse 84; temperature 99.5°; bowels moved by medicine. To have thirty grains of salicin every four hours.

29th.—Restless night; to-day he feels very wretched, especially as he cannot move; both ankles swollen and tender; knees less so; pulse 88; temperature 100.5°; bowels confined. To have half an ounce of castor oil; continue salicin.

30th.—Did not sleep well, but thinks he feels better; complains chiefly of inability to move his legs; joints unchanged in appearance, but evidently causing less pain; skin covered with acid perspiration; pulse 96; temperature 100.5°; bowels moved.

31st.—Had decidedly less pain during the night, but did not sleep much; to-day feels weaker, but is not in pain, and looks more cheerful; swelling almost gone from joints, which can now be handled without pain; can move right leg pretty freely; has pain in left arm, between shoulder and elbow but not affecting either joint; pulse 92; temperature 101.1°. Continue salicin.

Jan 1st.—Quiet night; pain and swelling gone from joints; has aching in muscles about shoulders; feels much better, and has desire for food; has much acid perspiration, of which he complains more than he does of pain; tongue cleaner; pulse 84; temperature 101.4°.

2nd.—Feels better; still muscular pain in left arm, but nowhere else; pulse 84; temperature 100.1°; takes food with relish. Continue salicin.

3rd.—Good night; no pain; pulse 76; temperature 99.8°.

4th.—Quiet night; free from pain; pulse 60; temp. 99°.

5th.—Ditto, ditto; pulse 56; temp. 98.2°. Remained well.

CASE 7.—James R——. aged forty-four. Has had rheumatic fever three or four times, lasting on each occasion from three to six weeks. Two days ago felt that his old enemy was returning.

Dec. 31st.—Has anxious expression; skin perspiring freely, acid reaction; tongue moist and furred; both knees painful, but not swollen; right wrist and fingers of both hands swollen and tender; has a soft (probably old) systolic murmur at apex; pulse 96; temperature 99°; bowels open. To have fifteen grains of salicin every three hours.

Jan. 1st.—Bad night; great pain in wrists; knees not so bad; profuse acid perspiration; pulse 96; temperature 99.9°. Continue salicin.

3rd.—Good night; no pain, only stiffness in affected joints, which are still somewhat swollen; pulse 92; temperature 98.8°.

4th.—Pain all gone; skin natural; cardiac murmur unchanged; pulse 88; temperature 98.5°.

Improvement continued. Said that nothing ever did him so much good as the powders, and that he never got over an attack so quickly.

CASE 8. *Chronic rheumatism.*—Alexander L——,, aged forty-five, married, was, four years ago, confined to the house for four months with rheumatism. Two years ago he was laid up in the same way for six weeks. On neither occasion were the joints affected, the pain being seated in the muscles and bones. Three weeks ago his old symptoms recurred rather suddenly, and have continued. During this time, under medical advice, he has been taking various salts of potsss, but without the least benefit.

Dec. 1st.—Complains of pain in back and limbs, much increased by any movement; has not got beyond the chair at the side of his bed for three weeks, and that he gets into with great difficulty; skin natural; tongue clean; bowels constipated; pulse 68, feeble; temperature 99°; heart-sounds normal. To have an aperient, and thirty grains of salicin every six hours.

3rd.—Not seen yesterday. Slept better last night than he has done for some time; feels decidedly better. His wife states that he is more cheerful than he has been for weeks; pains not so severe; pulse 68; temperature 98.4°.

5th.—Feels much better; can move about the house freely, having only slight pain in the lumbar region and in the left leg; pulse 68; temperature 98.2°. To have fifteen grains of salicin every four hours.

He continued to improve for some six weeks after leaving off the salicin, when his symptoms returned as badly as before, and this time accompanied by pain and swelling of right wrist. Took the powders of his own accord, and was at work again in a week. Says that nothing ever did him so much good as the powders.

The accompanying charts will show at a glance the daily range of temperature and rate of pulse in the seven cases of acute and subacute rhumatism which have been given. The continuous white lines indicate the temperature, the dotted lines the pulse.

From an examination of these charts alone, especially of the first four, one would almost certainly conclude that they indicated the ranges of temperature and pulse of so many cases of febricula, so rapid and so decided is the diminution of fever which followed the administration of the salicin. A perusal of the details of the cases, however, indicates their true nature. So much febrile disturbance, accompanied by pain and swelling of joints and profuse acid perspiration, form a combination of symptoms which nothing but the rheumatic poison could produce. The sudden arrest of the painful symptoms, and the coincident rapid fall of pulse and temperature, followed so immediately on the administration of the salicin that it is impossible not to attribute them to its use. Cases of acute rheumatism do sometimes improve in the most unexpected manner, but I never saw a case get well so quickly as those of which I have given details above. A succession of such cases cannot but be attributed to the peculiarity of the treatment. We have seen that this treatment has a good foundation in reason and analogy. The details of these cases af-

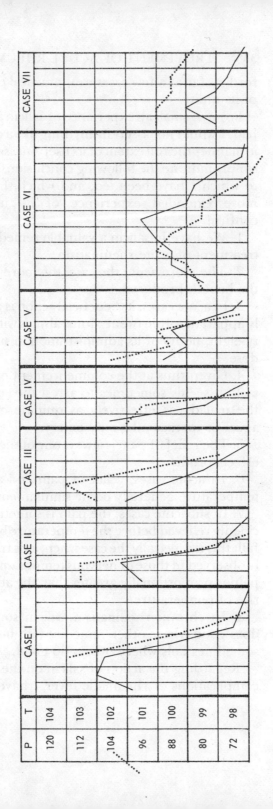

P	T
120	104
112	103
104	102
96	101
88	100
80	99
72	98

ford, as far as a few cases can, practical evidence of its utility.

From so small an experience of salicin as I have had, I would not assert in anything like a dogmatic manner the full extent of its usefulness. I would simply indicate the following conclusions as those to which I have been led, and which, I hope, a more extended experience of its use may confirm.

1. We have in salicin a valuable remedy in the treatment of acute rheumatism.

2. The more acute the case, the more marked the benefit produced.

3. In acute cases, its beneficial action is generally apparent within twenty-four, always within forty-eight, hours of its administration in sufficient dose.

4. Given thus at the commencement of the attack, it seems sometimes to arrest the course of the malady as effectively as quinine cures an ague, or ipecacuanha a dysentery.

5. The relief of pain is always one of the earliest effects produced.

6. In acute cases, relief of pain and a fall of temperature generally occur simultaneously.

7. In subacute cases, the pain is sometimes decidedly relieved before the temperature begins to fall; this is especially the case when, as is frequently observed in those of nervous temperament, the pain is proportionally greater than the abnormal rise of temperature.

8. In chronic rheumatism, salicin sometimes does good where other remedies fail; but it also sometimes fails where others do good.

Regarding the action of salicin on the cardiac complications of rheumatic fever I have no experience. In Case 1, indeed, the muffled and indistinct character of the heart's sounds, which existed before its administration, disappeared with the general improvement which accompanied its use. But it needs not the details of cases to demonstrate that a remedy which curtails the duration, or mitigates the severity, of an attack of rheumatic fever, must of necessity diminish in a proportionate degree the risk of cardiac mischief. Neither is it doubtful that the general treatment most suited for rheumatic endo- or peri-carditis is that which most surely and speedily cures the rheumatism. Rheumatic inflammation about the heart requires the same general treatment as rheumatic inflammation of a joint.

The dose of salicin is from ten to thirty grains every two, three, or four hours, according to the severity of the case. Fifteen grains every three hours is a medium dose for an acute case. It is very possible that less might suffice; for I have not tried to find the minimum dose. It is very certain that a much larger dose may be given without producing discomfort.

Salicin is not soluble to any useful extent; it is best administered as a powder mixed with a little cold water. It is a very pleasant bitter. I have never found the least inconvenience follow its use.

When salicylic acid (originally prepared from salicin) was first introduced, I determined to try it; and in the one case in which I did have recourse to it, it seemed to do good to the rheumatism; but it caused so much irritation of the throat and stomach that I did not repeat it. This was, no doubt, due to its being impure; for Traube has lately been trying it in his wards at Berlin, and reports most favourably as to its action in rheumatic fever.*

It is the publication of these observations that has led me to give to the profession so soon my favourable and prior experience of salicin in the same disease.

I have no doubt that Traube's observations are correct, and that salicylic acid will be found efficacious in the treatment of acute rheumatism. But I have as little doubt that it is not so good as salicin for this purpose; for it is more apt to contain noxious impurities, it is not so pleasant to take, and it apparently requires a larger dose to produce its beneficial action.

I shall be greatly obliged if those who try the remedy, and do not care to publish their observations, would kindly forward to me the results of their experience, be it favourable or otherwise. The points to be specially noted are the state of the patient, before taking the salicin, as regards heart, pulse, temperature, skin, tongue, urine, joints, &c., with daily (or more frequent) observations of the same points while under its influence. Observations taken only once a day, to be taken as nearly as possible at the same time on each day.

Dundee.

NOTES

*Aitken's Practice of Medicine, sixth edition, vol. i., p. 819.
†Dr. Garrod in Reynolds's System of Medicine, vol. i., p. 906.